Tables of contents

INTRODUCTION

A. History's whispers:

Part 1

Chapter 1

Chapter 2

Chapter 3

Chapter 4

Ingredients:

Find your balance:

Chapter 5

Safety precautions:

Bonus tip:

Temperature issues:

Chapter 6

1. A step-by-step guide to fermentation:

Fermentation principles:

- Microbial diversity:

2. Embark on a Fermentation Journey:

Chapter 7

For oily skin:

For dry skin:

Part 3

Chapter 8

Chapter 9

1.From Attic to Shine:

2.The Rice Water Revolution:

Happy Bath Bonus:

Chapter 10

Harmonious hair:
Say goodbye to split ends:

1.From grain to glory:

Dandruff treatment:

Part 4

Chapter 11

Upcycle:

Chapter 12

Conclusion

INTRODUCTION

Step-by-Step Guide to Extracting Rice Water for Skin:

"Unlock the Power of Rice Water: Your Essential Guide to Glowing Skin"

From grain to radiance: Revealing the rice water ritual for radiant skin Forget about fairy godmothers and magic potions.

The secret to radiant skin may just be found in your pantry, hidden among the grains of rice.

Rice water, a centuries-old Asian beauty secret, is growing in popularity thanks to its ability to transform dull skin into wet dreams.

But navigating the world of rice water extraction can be confusing, leaving you wondering: Is it brown or white?

Soak or ferment?

Don't worry, put down the stove and rice cooker!

This step-by-step guide to rice water extract for skin is your passport to clearer, brighter, more hydrated skin.

Forget the conflicting advice on the internet and take a practical, step-by-step approach designed for every skin type and comfort level.

Inside you'll find: The science behind the shine: Delve into the fascinating history of rice water and reveal the scientific reasons why it can work wonders for your skin your skin.

From hydration heroes to antioxidant allies, discover the hidden magic in every grain.

Choose your rice adventure: Brown, white, black, fermented?

We explore different types of rice water and their unique benefits, helping you find the perfect one for your skin's specific needs.

Unlock aquatic treasures: Let go of uncertainty!

This guide provides clear and concise instructions on different extraction methods, from simple maceration to trendy fermentation processes.

You'll quickly become a rice water expert!

More than just rinsing: Explore the exciting world of rice water applications.

From DIY face masks to skin-soothing toners, we'll show you how to incorporate rice water into your existing skin care routine for maximum results.

Safety first, shine second: We put your health first.

Learn about the potential risks and precautions you should take to ensure a safe and effective rice water journey for your unique skin.

This book is more than just a cookbook; it is an invitation to adopt a conscious and sustainable approach to beauty.

By harnessing the power of a natural ingredient, you'll not only nourish your skin, but also minimise waste and connect with ancient beauty traditions.

So grab your rice, unleash your inner alchemist and begin your journey towards radiant skin, one grain at a time!

From Rice Fields to Porcelain Skin: Revealing the Legacy of Rice Water Rice water, the newest buzzword in the world of skin care, may seem like just a fad, but its history goes far beyond glossy magazine pages.

It's a story passed down through generations, echoing from the misty rice fields of Asia to your modern bathroom counter.

Buckle up, beauty explorers, as we delve into the fascinating history and cultural significance of this seemingly simple body of water.

Picture this: centuries ago, women from China and Japan, with skin as smooth and bright as porcelain, knelt beside rice fields, collecting water left over from washing the grain.
It's not just water; it is a sacred elixir, imbued with the essence of life.
They intuitively knew what science would later confirm: rice water is the key to radiant skin.

A. History's whispers: Heian period in Japan: Legend has it that court ladies used rice water to wash their faces, attributing their youthful skin to its special properties.

its nurturing properties.

Tang Dynasty China: Bathing in rice water was considered a beauty ritual for concubines, whose skin was as soft as silk after immersing themselves in this milky treasure.

Southeast Asian Village: Even today, women in rural areas still use rice water to wash their faces and hair, preserving their natural beauty according to this time-tested tradition.

Cultural significance revealed: Respect for nature: Rice, the staple food, is revered as a gift from the earth.
Using water for beauty is considered a way to honour the generosity of nature.
Connect to the community: recipes and rituals for using rice water is a way for women to bond and pass down beauty secrets through generations.
Holistic approach: Rice water has more than just external beautifying effects; it is considered a way to nourish the body and mind, reflecting a holistic vision of well-being. Modern version: Today, science is catching up with ancient wisdom. Studies show that rice water can provide:

Increase hydration: Rich in starch and amino acids, helps lock in moisture, leaving skin plump and moisturized. Soothing properties: Its soothing and anti-inflammatory nature can soothe irritation and redness.
Brightening Benefits: Some believe it can gently exfoliate, resulting in brighter, more radiant skin. But remember that cultural appropriation is never pretty.

While appreciating the wisdom of the past, remember to do so with respect, recognizing the origins and honouring the traditions behind this ancient beauty method. So, next time you pick up that bowl of rice, remember that within those tiny grains of rice lies a legacy of beauty waiting to be revealed.

Explore the world of rice water but respect its history and cultural significance. Your skin may thank you and your journey will be even more rewarding.

B. Rice water rhapsody: A symphony of skin benefits (but still guaranteed!) Rice water, the newest beauty product, has skin care enthusiasts humming with hope.

But before you throw out your favourite serum and replace it with a bowl of rice soak, let's dive into the science (and add a little healthy scepticism) to understand its potential, not its promises. its appointment. Picture this: a shimmering waterfall of rice, washing away not only the grains but also the centuries-old folklore of its skin-friendly magic.

Although research is still in the early stages, some potential benefits have emerged, such as Wind Whispers: Hydration Hero: Rice water is rich in starch, which can act as a moisturizer, Attracts and locks in moisture, making your skin smoother. plump and moist.

Think of it like a sponge that absorbs water and keeps your skin hydrated and plump. Soothing Serenade: Some studies show that rice water may have mild anti-inflammatory properties, potentially soothing irritation and redness. Think of it as a gentle lullaby for your skin, soothing any discomfort.

Brightening Bonanza: Rice water may contain ferric acid, an antioxidant that some believe helps fight free radicals and generally brighten skin tone. Imagine the sun peeking through the clouds, revealing a lighter, more radiant person. However, remember that beauty is not a fairy tale:

Not guaranteed: While these potential benefits are promising, they are not guaranteed for everyone. Skin types vary and what works wonders for one person may fail for another. Don't expect an overnight transformation; Think of it as a gentle melody, not a dramatic symphony.

Limited Research: Most studies on the effects of rice water on the skin are small-scale or preliminary. Further research is needed to fully understand its impact and long-term effectiveness. Think of this as a work in progress, not a finished masterpiece.

Quality issues: Not all rice water is equal. The type of rice, soaking method, and storage all affect the characteristics of the rice. Pay attention to supplies and preparation to ensure you get the right things. So should you give up your current habit to perform the ritual of drinking rice water? Unnecessary.

But if you're curious and enjoy exploring natural ingredients, it might be worth a try. Remember, approach it with an open mind, realistic expectations, and a healthy dose of research. Ultimately, the most beautiful symphony is the one your skin plays. Listen to their needs, experiment carefully, and find what works best for your unique creation. After all, true beauty must shine from within and that is a tone that no amount of rice water can replace.

C. get caught up in the hype: Exposing the Ritual of Rice Water Rice water, the newest favorite skin care product, has taken the beauty world by storm. But amid the glowing testimonials and rave reviews, it's easy to get swept away with the flow. Before you ditch the serum and invest in a lifetime supply of rice, let's dive into the murky waters of common misconceptions and limitations surrounding this trendy ingredient.

Misconception #1: Rice water is a miracle drug: Imagine this: Just a bowl of rice water will turn your skin into porcelain overnight. Unfortunately, the reality is less magical. Although rice water is promising, its benefits are not miraculous. Moisturizing, soothing, and brightening effects are potential, not guaranteed, and will vary greatly depending on your skin type and specific preparation method.

Misconception #2: All rice water is created equal: Not really. The type of rice, soaking method and storage time all affect the rice's properties. Brown rice water contains more antioxidants, while fermented rice water may provide more benefits. But remember, just like rice, not all versions are created equal. Research your options and choose wisely.

Misconception #3: Ditch everything else: Save your serum! Rice water is not the only solution for skin care. It can supplement your current routine but can't replace everything else you're using. Think of it as a sweet melody, not the entire symphony of your skincare routine.

Limitation #1: Research limitation: Although studies are ongoing, scientific evidence for the effectiveness of rice water is still in its early stages. Further research is needed to fully understand its impact and long-term effectiveness on different skin types. Remember that beauty trends often go beyond scientific confirmation.

Limitation #2: Individual differences: What is magical for one person may make another person's skin less radiant. Listen to your skin and don't be afraid to experiment with caution. If you experience irritation, skip the rice and consult a dermatologist. So should we throw away the bowl of rice water? Unnecessary.

If you are curious and enjoy exploring natural ingredients then it may be worth a try. Remember, approach it with realistic expectations, do your research, and prioritise your skin health above all else. Ultimately, the most beautiful light comes from within and from wise choices. Don't get caught up in the hype; Explore rice water carefully and find what best suits your skin's unique story. After all, the most attractive beauty is the one that truly shines.

Part 1

Delving into the galaxy: Revealing the mysteries of rice water for skin Rice water, the newest beauty buzzword, can be found on your bathroom counter just like a mysterious parchment. Is it a miracle drug that promises porcelain-white skin, or just another fad that will fade? Fear not, intrepid explorer of beauty, for we are about to embark on a journey to decode the truth hidden in this milky treasure.

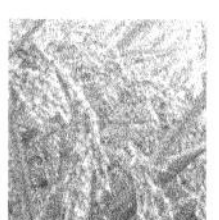

This image: sunny rice fields swaying gently, each grain of rice holds the potential for radiant skin. Legends whisper that ancient Asian cultures used rice water for beauty purposes, but what lies beneath the mysterious surface of this milk?

Enter the Lab: Hydration Hero: Rice water is rich in starch, acting like a sponge, absorbing and retaining moisture, making the skin plump and moisturised. Think of it as a gentle rain that nourishes the parched earth.

Soothing Serenade: Some studies show that its anti-inflammatory properties can soothe irritation and redness, providing a soothing tone to sensitive skin. Imagine a soothing lullaby for your skin.

Brightening Bonanza: Rice water may contain ferulic acid, an antioxidant that some believe helps fight free radicals and brighten the skin. Think of it like sunlight breaking through the clouds, revealing a lighter, more radiant self.

But wait, beauty explorer: No Fairy Godmother: While these potential benefits are enticing, they are not guaranteed. Individual differences prevail and what works for one person may make another person's skin less happy. Remember that beauty is a unique journey, not a unique fairy tale.

Limited Research: The science of rice water is still in its infancy, like a half-written scroll. Further studies are needed to fully understand its impact and long-term effectiveness on different skin types. Be aware of the hype and research reliable information before jumping in.

Quality issues: Not all rice water is equal. The type of rice, soaking method, and storage all affect the characteristics of the rice. Think of it like choosing the right brush for your masterpiece – quality matters! So should you give up your current habit of bathing in rice water? Unnecessary.

But if you're curious and enjoy exploring natural ingredients, this could be a worthwhile adventure. Remember: Approach with caution: Start slowly, test your skin and listen to your skin.

This is not a medicine to swallow; it is a delicate experience that requires observation and care. Do your research: Dive into the science, understand the limitations, and explore different preparation methods. Be your own beauty detective, not a blind trend follower.

Celebrate your uniqueness: There is no one way to achieve radiant skin. Show off your personality, experiment thoughtfully, and find what works best for your unique layout. Ultimately, the most beautiful light comes from within and from wise choices. Don't be swayed by the hype; Explore rice water carefully and let your own skin story unfold. Remember that the sexiest beauty is the one that shines authentically, has a little curiosity and a lot of friends.

Chapter 1

1.Unmasking the dairy maze: Navigating the diverse world of rice water Rice water, the newest beauty elixir, beckons us like a shimmering oasis in a desert of care trends skin. But before you begin, remember that not all rice water is created equal. Each, like a grain in the field, has its own properties and potential benefits. So, grab your magnifying glass, beauty explorer, and let's dive into the diverse world of this dairy treasure:

Colour Chronicles:

Brown Rice Water: This earthly warrior, Full of antioxidants and minerals, it may be your best choice. to fight free radicals and promote healthy, glowing skin. Think of it as a shield against harmful environmental factors, keeping your skin healthy and elastic.

White Rice Water: This gentle soul drink, rich in starch and amino acids, is known for its super moisturising properties. Think of it as a plumping shot, leaving your skin as dewy and soft as a freshly steamed rice cake.

Black Rice Water: This rare gem, rich in anthocyanins and antioxidants, may provide anti-inflammatory and skin-soothing properties. Think of it as a gentle balm, capable of reducing redness and irritation.

Fermented factor: Unfermented: This classic choice retains its natural properties, offering a simple approach to enjoying the benefits of rice water. Think of it as a familiar, comforting, and trustworthy tune.

Fermentation: This experimental elixir undergoes a transformation process, potentially increasing antioxidant content and providing additional skin benefits. Think of it as a fun version that adds a unique touch to the rice water experience. Remember, the perfect rice water is as unique as you are:

Consider your skin type: Sensitive skin may prefer gentle white rice water, while oily skin may benefit from the Astringent properties of black rice water. Listen to your skin's needs and choose accordingly.

Don't follow trends: Although fermented rice water is trendy, it may not be necessary for everyone. Explore the different types and see which one is right for your skin.

Quality issues: Buy rice wisely and make sure to prepare it well. Contaminated rice water can do more harm than good. So, start your rice water journey with an open mind and clear eyes.

Experiment with caution, research the different types and choose the one that best fits your unique skin story. Remember, the best lighting comes from wise choices and a little exploration.

After all, the most captivating beauty is the true radiance of beauty, sprinkled with the magic of rice water, if that's your cup of tea!

1. The Rice Rumble: White vs. Brown, Long vs. Short - A Cereal Showdown for Beauty Lovers Rice Water, the newest skin care favourite, takes us to the first world of this versatile grain.

But before you get lost in the milk maze, let's settle a debate older than time: white versus brown and long versus short. Hold on to your spoons, beauty adventurers, because this rice dish is about to get delicious (and informative)!

White rice vs. brown rice: Nutritional face-off **White rice:** Refined Prince, which removes the bran and germ, has a softer texture and cooks faster. But like a charming thug, it lacks the fibre and nutrients contained in these extracted parts. Think of it as beauty without substance (at least in the nutritional sense).

Brown Rice: Earthy Warrior is whole grain, unprocessed, high in fibre, vitamins and minerals. It may not be as tender or cook as quickly as the white variety, but its nutritional value is very high. Think of it as a powerful hero, providing lasting benefits to your skin and overall health.

Grain or Short Grain: Tango Texture Long Grain Rice: Independent Dancer, known for its fine, separated grains, cooks tenderly and does not clump easily. Think of it as a light and airy waltz that hits your taste buds (and maybe your skin).

Short Grain Rice : This sticky rice, known for its sticky, chewy grains, creates a creamy texture perfect for sushi and risotto. Think of it as a passionate tango, leaving its mark on your dish (and ultimately your rice water).

Now the million dollar question: who will win the rice water crown?
Depending on personal preference and your skin type:
For pure moisturizing: White rice water can be a good choice due to its starch content.

For nutritional supplements: Brown rice water offers a more comprehensive approach to fiber and vitamins.
For sensitive skin: Long grain rice water may be gentler due to its lower starch nature.

For a thicker consistency: Short-grain rice water may be ideal if you prefer a richer, creamier texture. Remember that the most beautiful rice water is the rice water that suits you.

Experiment, listen to your skin and don't be afraid to mix & match to create the perfect beauty elixir for yourself. After all, the sexiest glow comes from accepting your unique needs and finding what makes your skin sing (and dance, maybe a tango?).

So, grab your rice cooker, unleash your inner alchemist and start your journey to radiant skin, one grain at a time!

2. Fermentation showdown: The acidic transformation of rice water Rice water, the rising star of skin care, has many faces. Today we dive into the ancient art of fermentation, a process that turns this simple water into a potentially powerful elixir. But is it worth the wait? Buckle up, beauty adventurers, because the fermenting face-off is about to get frothy!

Classic Competitor: Unfermented Rice Water Simple: This pure version retains the natural properties of rice, providing hydration and soothing properties. Think of it as a gentle, familiar, and comforting melody. Quick and easy: No waiting game here! Simply soak the rice and reap the results immediately.

It's like instant gratification for your skin. Soft and gentle: Non-fermented means less risk of irritation, making it a good choice for those with sensitive souls. Think of it as a soothing lullaby for your skin. Tested Elixir:

Fermented Rice Water Sour Metabolism: Fermentation introduces good bacteria, which has the potential to increase antioxidant content and provide additional skin benefits. Think of it as a fun version that adds a unique touch to the rice water experience.

Potential potency: studies show that fermented rice water can provide anti-aging and skin-brightening properties, like a miracle drug for youthful-looking skin. Think of it as a symphony of benefits waiting to be discovered. Patience is a virtue:

Fermentation takes time, requiring planning and waiting. It's like a love story that unfolds slowly, building anticipation with potential payoffs. But wait, beauty alchemists!
Before you get the fermentation kit: Not the magic potion: Both versions have limitations. Research is still ongoing and results may vary depending on your skin type. Remember that beauty is not a fairy tale.

Quality is important: Ensure good hygiene and use clean ingredients. Contaminated rice water can do more harm than good. Don't prepare for disaster in the name of beauty!
Listen to your skin: Start slowly, do a patch test, and see how your skin reacts. Each outfit is a unique story and what suits one person may not suit another. So who wins in the fermentation showdown?

The answer lies right within you! Consider your skin type, patience level, and desired benefits. Experiment responsibly and find the version of rice water that best highlights your unique beauty story. After all, the most captivating brilliance comes from wise choices and a little exploration. So go ahead, beauty adventurers, and let your skin.

Chapter 2

Delving into the Rice Fields' pantry: Revealing the science behind Rice Water's skin secrets, Rice water, the newest beauty elixir, has captivated skincare enthusiasts Skincare with whispers of ancient wisdom and promises of radiant skin. But behind this fascinating folklore lies a world of science waiting to be discovered. So, with your magnifying glass, beauty detectives, let's dive into the fascinating world of active ingredients and their potential benefits for the skin!

Discover the treasure: Carbs: This humble carbohydrate acts like a sponge, attracting and holding moisture, leaving your skin plump and dewy. Think of it as a microscopic reservoir, keeping your skin hydrated and plump.

Amino Acids: These protein building blocks can help strengthen the skin barrier, improving its resilience and texture. Think of them as tiny architects working tirelessly to strengthen your skin's protective wall.

Antioxidants: Fermented rice water contains warriors such as ferulic acid, which has the ability to fight free radicals and delay signs of aging. Think of them as shields that repel harmful environmental factors, keeping your skin youthful.

Vitamins and Minerals: Brown rice water provides a treasure trove of these micronutrients, which have the ability to support skin health and give it a healthy glow. Think of them as the vitamins your skin needs, nourishing it from the inside out. But hold your horses, you beauty alchemists!

The science is still in its early stages: Limited research: Although these studies are promising, more research is needed to fully understand and confirm the long-term effects of rice water on different skin types. Pay attention to the hype and rely on reliable sources.

Individual Differences: What works wonders for one person may leave another person's skin less delighted. Remember that your skin is unique and so are its needs. Listen carefully and test carefully.

No guarantees: Although the science is promising, it does not guarantee results. Think of it as a potential ally in your skin care journey, not a panacea. So should you give up your current habit of bathing in rice water? Unnecessary! But if you're curious and enjoy exploring natural ingredients, it might be worth a try. Remember:

Approach with caution: Start slowly, try a patch and see how your skin reacts. This is not a medicine to swallow; it is a delicate experience that requires careful observation. Research is key: Dive into the science, understand the limitations, and explore different preparation methods.

Be your own beauty detective, not a blind trend follower. Celebrate your uniqueness: There is no one way to achieve radiant skin. Show off your personality, experiment thoughtfully, and find what works best for your unique layout.

Ultimately, the most beautiful light comes from within and from wise choices. Don't be swayed by the hype; Explore rice water carefully and let your own skin story unfold. Remember that the sexiest beauty is the one that shines authentically, has a little curiosity and a lot of friends.

1 Beauty Bodybuilders: Vitamins, Minerals and Amino Acids - The Foundation of Radiant Skin Imagine your skin as a beautiful city, thriving thanks to the contributions of its residents. Just like busy citizens, small molecules called vitamins, minerals and amino acids play an important role in keeping your skin healthy and bright.
So, buckle up, beauty architects, and let's embark on a journey to understand these microscopic wonders!

Vitamins: Essential substances: Vitamin A (Retinol): This super skin care product helps fight wrinkles and stimulates collagen production, giving you firmer, smoother skin. Think of it as a team of construction workers, rebuilding your skin's scaffolding for youthful-looking skin.

Vitamin C: This antioxidant warrior protects your skin from free radicals, the bad guys that cause premature ageing. Think of it as an army of little soldiers, deflecting harmful rays and protecting your skin.

Vitamin E: This hydrating hero locks in moisture, leaving your skin soft and supple. Think of it as a team of professional gardeners, nurturing your skin's delicate ecosystem and keeping it well-watered.

Minerals: Powerful Micronutrients: Zinc: This powerful anti-inflammatory helps calm redness and irritation, leaving your skin feeling soothed and balanced. Think of it as a fire brigade, extinguishing any flare-ups and maintaining your skin's peace.

Selenium: This antioxidant ally works alongside vitamin E to fight free radicals and protect your skin from damage. Think of them as a dynamic duo, fighting against ageing and keeping your skin healthy.

Magnesium: This relaxing maestro helps regulate sebum production, keeping your skin clear and balanced. Think of it as a team of Zen masters, calming chaos and promoting harmony in your pores.
Amino Acids: Beauty Ingredients: Arginine: This amino acid helps produce collagen, the protein that gives your skin its elasticity and elasticity. Think of it as a team of masons, building the foundation for your skin's youthful structure.

Tyrosine: This melanin-producing maestro helps determine your skin tone and protects it from harmful UV rays. Think of it as a team of artists, giving your skin a healthy glow and providing natural protection.
Glycine: This moisturising hero promotes collagen production and helps maintain your skin's moisture. Think of it as a team of water bearers, ensuring your skin stays plump and dewy. Remember that beauty thrives on synergy: A healthy diet rich in fruits, vegetables and whole grains provides your body with the building blocks needed to make these essential nutrients.
Think of it as nurturing the soil so your beauty can flourish. Consult your doctor: Individual needs vary and supplements may sometimes be needed. Seek expert advice to ensure you get what your skin really needs. Listen to your skin: Experiment with different foods and see how your skin reacts.

Every skin tone has its own story and what works for one person may not work for another. So unleash the architect of your inner beauty! By understanding the important role of vitamins, minerals and amino acids, you can help your skin glow from the inside out.

Remember, true beauty radiates from a healthy foundation, nurtured by wise choices and self-discovery. So, build your beautiful city brick by brick and let your radiant personality shine!

Antioxidant army: Little warriors guarding your skin's fortress Imagine your skin as a magnificent castle, constantly besieged by free radicals and harmful substances. Toxic molecules destroy its youthful beauty. But fear not, beauty warriors! Nature has given you a mighty army of antioxidants, tiny shields against these invisible enemies.

Let's dive into the fascinating world of these skin care superheroes and their potential impact on your skin health. Antioxidants: Beauty guardian angels: radicals' enemies: Free radicals, like rogue robbers, damage the collagen and elasticity in your skin, leading to wrinkles, loss of firmness, and a dull appearance.

Antioxidants, like brave knights, neutralise these villains, thereby preserving the youthful structure of your skin.

Solar Shield Soldiers: Exposure to sunlight is the main source of free radicals. Antioxidants, which act as sun warriors, provide extra protection, minimising damage caused by harmful UV rays, keeping your skin healthy and glowing. **Anti-inflammatory**: Inflammation, another beauty enemy, can lead to redness, irritation and even premature ageing.

Antioxidants promote their ability to soothe your skin, reduce inflammation and promote healthy, balanced skin. But remember that even heroes have limits: Not all antioxidants are equal: Different antioxidants offer different levels of protection and target different specific free radicals. Research and select a diverse team of antioxidant heroes for optimal defence.

The diet plays an important role: Your body naturally produces some antioxidants, but dietary sources such as fruits, vegetables and whole grains are essential for nourishment. Energise your army. Nourish your skin from within!

Individual needs vary: Like a personalised defence strategy, your skin's specific needs will determine your antioxidant choice. Consult a dermatologist to get expert advice on tailoring your skin care arsenal. So should you ditch the sunscreen and rely solely on antioxidants?

Insufficient. Antioxidants are powerful allies, but sunscreen is still your first line of defence against sun damage. Think of them as complementary forces, working together to protect your skin's fortress. Ultimately, the best glowing skin comes from a holistic approach:

Adopting a healthy lifestyle: Nourishing your body with a balanced diet, regular exercise and adequate sleep will strengthen your skin's natural defences, allowing your antioxidant army to work more effectively.

Explore different options: From topical skin care products to dietary choices, research and test different antioxidant sources to find the one that best suits your needs.

Celebrate your personality: Every skin tells a unique story. Listen to its needs, exploit its strengths and give it the means to shine naturally, with the help of your brave army of antioxidants. Remember that true beauty radiates from within, nurtured by wise choices and a little self-discovery. So arm your skin with the power of antioxidants and let your radiant self conquer the world, one free radical at a time!

Chapter 3

The Rice Fields: Safety Beacons for Your Rice Water Journey Rice water, the newest beauty product, beckons with the promise of radiant skin. But before we dive headfirst into this milky wonderland, let's sound the safety bell and shed light on potential risks and considerations. Remember that beauty should not be exchanged for happiness!

Potential Pitfalls: Contamination Caper: Poor hygiene or using unclean rice can introduce bacteria or toxins, leading to irritation, infection or worse. Think of it as a murky pond, containing unpredictable dangers. Unexpected realisation: Even natural ingredients can cause allergies or sensitivities.

Start by examining your skin and carefully observing its reaction. Remember that even the gentlest giant can trip you up. Individuality Ignored: Not all leather is created equal. What is miraculous to one person may be less than joyful to another. Listen to your skin's unique voice and adjust accordingly.

Safety Card: Hygiene Hero: Always use clean, filtered water and wash rice thoroughly before soaking. Think of it like sterilising your tools before embarking on your beauty routine.

Quality Matters: Choose organic rice whenever possible to minimise exposure to pesticides or chemicals. Remember, the purity of your ingredients matters!

Start slow and easy: Start with diluted rice water and gradually increase the concentration as your skin adapts. This is a marathon, not a sprint, so use gentle exploration for a quick fix.

Listen to your skin: Pay close attention to any signs of irritation, redness or discomfort. If any problems occur, stop using immediately and consult a dermatologist. Your skin is the ultimate guide, so follow its advice as Your true beauty thrives on wise choices:

Research Is your guide. Dig into trusted sources, learn the science behind rice water, and avoid becoming a victim of sensational claims. Knowledge is power, beauty exploration!

Expert advice is essential: If you have any pre-existing skin conditions or problems, seek advice from a dermatologist before incorporating rice water into your routine. Let the experts navigate this difficult terrain.

Take a holistic approach: Nourishing your body with a healthy diet, managing stress and getting enough sleep will contribute greatly to your overall health and glowing skin. Beauty flourishes from within, so maintain the entire garden. So should you give up your current habit to perform the ritual of drinking rice water?

Unnecessary. But if you're curious and interested in exploring natural ingredients, approach them with a cautious heart, a clear eye, and a commitment to safety. Let your journey into rice water be a mindful exploration rather than a reckless plunge. Ultimately, the most beautiful light comes from within and shines through wise choices.

Remember, self-love and acceptance are the real secrets of beauty. So explore rice water responsibly, celebrate your skin's unique story, and let your inner light shine!

1.Explore the skin maze: Patch tests your path to radiant skin Imagine your skin as a living tapestry, woven with sensitive, bespoke threads for you.

Entering the new world of skin care, like rice water, can be exciting, but before you dive in, remember: Skin testing is your safe harbour for exploration. Let's dive into the fascinating world of skin sensitivity and discover the secrets of skin testing, the key to achieving radiant, worry-free skin.

Whispers of Sensitivity: Hidden Dragons: Did you know that certain ingredients, even natural ones, can cause hidden sensitivities, leading to rashes? redness, irritation or worse?

Think of them as sleeping dragons, waiting to be awakened by a bad touch.

The individual reigns supreme: What is miraculous to one person can leave another's skin like a battlefield. Your skin, like your fingerprints, is unique, so understanding its sensitivity is important. Patch test:

Your safety beacon: A small test, big results: Applying a small amount of product to a hidden area (usually behind the ear) will help your skin

Sleep Test: Your Safety Signal: A Small Test, Big Results: Apply a small amount of product to a hidden area (usually behind the ear) allowing your skin to whisper the feeling Real contact before taking full action.

Blowing adventure. Think of it as testing the waters before diving in. Listen carefully: Pay attention to any redness, itching, burning, or swelling within 24 to 48 hours. Even a small whisper can signal impending trouble.

Consult your dermatologist: If you experience any side effects, seek professional advice. They can help you decode the language of your skin and navigate the world of skin care safely. Remember that patch testing is not a one-time event:

New is not always better: Even products you have used before can cause sensitization in time. Patch testing is your faithful companion, always by your side to explore new horizons in skin care. As the seasons change, so does your skin:

Your skin's needs and sensitivities may fluctuate with the seasons. Regular patch testing ensures that you stay current with its ever-changing needs. Real beauty comes from wise choices and **self-love**: Appreciate your uniqueness: Don't compare your skin's reaction to the reaction of others. Honour their individuality and meet their specific needs using patch testing.

Knowledge is power: Dive into the science behind ingredients, look for hidden sensitivities, and prioritise safety over quick fixes. Remember, wise choices will pave the way to radiant skin.

Love your skin: Nourish your skin with a healthy diet, manage stress, and prioritise sleep. True beauty shines from within, so treat your skin with the love and respect it deserves. So, before starting your rice water journey, remember the power of skin testing.

It is your compass that will guide you through the complex maze of skin sensitivity. With a careful heart, a clear mind, and a commitment to self-love, you can discover the secret to radiant, healthy skin in just one safe exploration.

2.Rice Water Rhapsody: Hygiene and Conservation - The Unsung Heroes of Your Skin Symphony Rice Water, the new beauty muse, promises harmonious radiance. But before you unleash your inner alchemist, remember: the stage must be set!

Unhygienic practices and haphazard storage can turn your symphony of beauty into a jarring mess. So let's focus on the unsung heroes of your **skin care journey:** cleaning and care best practices!

Hygiene: Prelude to perfection Think like a chef: Imagine your rice water as a delicious dish. Do you use dirty utensils? Of course not! Wash the rice thoroughly before soaking and use filtered or boiled water to avoid unwanted guests from ruining your beauty evening.

Cleanliness is key: Wash your hands before handling rice and water, just like a conductor meticulously washes his baton before each performance. Remember that even the smallest contaminant can disrupt harmony.

Storage Containers Important: Choose a clean, airtight container to store rice water. Think of them as stylish displays for your cosmetic jar, protecting it from harmful elements like dust and bacteria.

Storage: The Encore for lasting beauty **Refrigerate your elixir:** Like a prized vintage, rice water thrives in the cool embrace of the refrigerator. This slows the growth of bacteria, ensuring your beauty potion stays fresh and lasts longer.

Tag love: Don't let your creativity become a forgotten mystery! Clearly label your rice water with the preparation date to avoid confusion or expired beauty products. Time is of the essence that even the most miraculous drugs have an expiration date. Use rice water within 2-3 days to ensure optimal results and avoid unwanted surprises.

Remember, true beauty is a holistic practice: Cleanliness goes beyond products: Nourish your body with healthy foods, manage stress and prioritise sleep. These contribute to healthy skin, creating a harmonious foundation for your rice water magic.

Listen to your skin: Every skin is unique. Observe how your skin reacts to rice water and adjust your workout accordingly. Remember that you are the conductor and your skin is the orchestra: create a melody that resonates within you.

Enjoy the journey: Embrace the process of discovering natural ingredients and creating your own skin care routines. Remember, the most beautiful light comes from a joyful heart and a commitment to self-care.

So, as you embark on your rice water adventure, remember: cleaning and storage are not just secondary but essential for perfect performance. With a little mindfulness and these best practices, you can create a harmonious skin symphony that will have everyone clapping!

PART 2

Rice Water Rhapsody: Reveals Extract Secrets and DIY Recipes Rice Water, the new muse of beauty, beckons with whispers of ancient wisdom and radiant skin. But before you unleash your inner alchemist, explore the different tones of extraction methods and develop some DIY recipes that suit your unique skin!

Extraction: Choose Your Tone Serenade Soak: This classic method gently extracts nutrients from rice, creating soft, versatile water. Think of it as a soothing lullaby, perfect for sensitive skin. Simply soak washed rice in filtered water for 30 minutes to an hour.

The Fermented Funk: This risky method infuses rice water with probiotics, potentially increasing its antioxidant content. Think of it as a fun improvisation, adding a unique touch to your beauty routine. Soak the rice for 24 to 48 hours, drain and let it ferment for another day or two.

The Boiled Ballad: This quick method releases more starch from the rice, giving it a thicker consistency. Think of it as a dramatic tone, perfect for dry skin. Boil washed rice for 15 minutes, filter and let cool before using.

DIY Recipe: Compose your beauty symphony Hydration Hero: Mix cooked rice water with a few drops of aloe vera gel to create a refreshing and hydrating mist. This simple formula is like a gentle rain for your skin.

Soothing Serenade: Mix rice water with a little honey to create a soothing mask that helps reduce redness and irritation. Think of it as a lullaby for your skin, soothing all discomforts.

Brightening Ball: Mix rice water with a few drops of lemon juice to create a skin-brightening toner, helping to even out skin tone.

This formula is like a ray of sunshine illuminating your skin. Remember that every skin is unique, so personalise your recipes: Experiment with ratios: Adjust amounts of rice and water to achieve desired consistency and richness . Remember that each tone needs its own balance.

Listen to your skin: Start with a diluted version and gradually increase the concentration as your skin adapts. Be your own conductor, listen carefully to your skin's preferences. Patch Test

Your Symphony: Before applying a formula to your entire face, test it on a small area to avoid any adverse reactions. Remember that discretion is the key to a harmonious beauty journey.

Beyond recipes: Holistic approach Nourish from within: Remember that beauty starts from within. Eat a healthy diet, manage stress, and prioritise sleep for a healthy foundation. Think of it like tuning your instrument before any performance.

Consult your dermatologist: If you have a pre-existing skin condition, seek expert advice before incorporating rice water into your routine. Let the experts harmonise your skin care symphony.

Embrace the journey: Enjoy the process of discovering natural ingredients and creating your own beauty rituals. Remember, the most radiant beauty comes from self-discovery and love for your unique skin. So, unleash your inner alchemist and embark on a rice water adventure!

With the right extraction methods, personalised recipes, and a mindful approach, you can create a symphony of beauty that leaves your skin radiant. Remember that the sexiest melody is always the one that resonates within you!

Chapter 4

Soaked Rice Music: Revealing the Simple Power of Rice Water Rice water, the new beauty muse, whispers the promise of radiant skin. But amid the swirling trends and complicated methods, there lurks a sweet melody: soaking methods. This simple, proven method provides a soothing lullaby to your skin, perfect for those looking for an accessible, natural path to beauty.

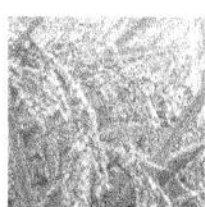

This image: sunny rice fields swaying gently, each grain of rice holds the potential to create a soothing symphony. The gentle soaking method transforms these precious nutrients into a milky elixir, ready to serve your skin. No complicated steps, no weird ingredients, just pure simplicity.

The enchanting melody of the soaking method: **Moisturizing hero:** Soaking rice water is rich in starch, acting like a sponge to absorb and retain moisture. Think of it as a gentle rain that nourishes your parched skin, leaving it plump and moisturised.

Soothing Serenade: Some studies show that its anti-inflammatory properties can soothe irritation and redness, providing a soothing tone to sensitive skin. Think of it as a lullaby for your skin, soothing all discomforts.

Simple Symphony: No fancy equipment, no lengthy procedures. Just steep, strain and enjoy the magic. This method is a wonderful ode to simplicity, perfect for busy lives and minimalist habits. But remember that every skin is unique,

So listen to its whispers: Start with a gentle tone: Start with diluted rice water and gradually increase the concentration as your skin likes it doubt. This is a progressive melody rather than a sudden explosion of sound.

Patch Test your Serenade: Before applying it to your entire face, test it on a small area to avoid any unwanted reactions. Remember that discretion is the key to a harmonious beauty journey. Don't be afraid to experiment:

Explore different soaking times, rice varieties, and even add a little honey for extra nutrition. Every skin has its own favourite rhythm, so find yours! Soaking method:

Simple introduction to beauty Nourishment from within: Remember that beauty starts from within. Eat a healthy diet, manage stress, and prioritise sleep for a healthy foundation. Think of it like tuning your instrument before any performance.

Listen to your skin: Pay attention to how your skin reacts. If you feel uncomfortable, adjust your approach or seek professional advice. Your skin is in charge, so follow its lead. Embrace the journey:

Enjoy the process of discovering natural ingredients and creating your own simple beauty ritual that has the most radiant beauty comes from self-discovery and love for your unique skin. So if you're looking for a gentle, accessible way to glowing skin, let soaking be your guide.

With its simple melody and gentle rhythm, it can become your skin's favourite lullaby, giving you a refreshing, soothing and beautiful feeling. Remember that the most captivating music is often the music that touches your unique soul.

1. Soothing symphony of soaking rice in water: Step-by-step instructions Imagine:

You are surrounded by a calm meadow, sunlight filtering through the wispy clouds, while a soundtrack softly echoed in the background. That's the feeling we're aiming for with soaking, a simple yet effective way to create nourishing rice water for your skin.

Ingredients: 1/2 cup uncooked rice (brown or white) 2-3 cups filtered water Bowl or pot with lid Fine mesh strainer Options:

Essential oils, aloe vera gel, honey

Step 1: Choose your melody (choose rice) Think of rice as the instrument of your beauty symphony. Brown rice provides a deeper, more earthy tone, while white rice provides a softer, more refined tone. Choose based on your preferences and skin type.

Step 2: Eliminate jitters (wash the rice) Like warming up before a performance, gently rinse the rice several times to remove dust or impurities. Think of it like cleaning your musical instrument for perfect performance.

Step 3: Set the Mood (Soak Time) This is where you create the duration of the melody. For a soothing lullaby, soak for 30 minutes. If you prefer a more intense look, aim for 1 to 2 hours. Remember that a longer soak will extract more starch, making the liquid thicker.

Step 4: Final step (Filter and preserve) Filter the rice water into a clean pot or bottle using a fine mesh strainer. Imagine separating the pure melody from the instrument.

Store rice water in the refrigerator for up to 3 days to ensure rice water is always fresh for your next beauty treatment.

Additional variations: Add a little honey for a soothing and hydrating mask. Mix a few drops of your favourite essential oil for personalised fragrance and potential skin benefits.
Use cooked rice water as rose water or cooling rose water. Remember that every skin is unique, **1.so listen to its whispers:**
Start with diluted rice water and gradually increase the concentration as your skin adapts. Patch test before applying to your entire face.

Enjoy the process of creating your own personalised beauty ritual. With this guide and a little creativity, you can turn a simple soak into a beautiful symphony for your skin! Now go ahead and create your own radiant tone!

2. Rice water decoded Recipe: Find the perfect harmony between grains and drops. Rice water, the new beauty muse, invites you with the promise of radiant skin. But amid the whirlwind of formulas and ratios, confusion still reigns.

Fear not, beauty adventurer! We will begin the journey to decode and discover the secrets to finding the perfect rice-water ratio, a harmonious blend for your unique skin.

Imagine this: a bustling market, overflowing with varieties of rice - the long, thin grains whisper tales of delicate hydration, the round, plump grains promise deeper nourishment . Together with them, water, an important element of beauty, is waiting for you in various forms:

filtered water, spring water, even soaked with herbs and spices. Ongoing mission? To create a harmonious blend, a symphony of grains and drops that express your skin's specific needs.

The Art of Alchemy in Scale: Basic Notes: Start with the basics - 1 cup uncooked rice. But here's the thing: each type of grain brings its own melody. Long grains like basmati or jasmine give a softer and more delicate feel, perfect for sensitive skin. Short-grain rice like sushi rice offers a richer, fuller experience, ideal for dry skin.

The Embrace of Water: From now on, water whispers its secrets. Filtered or spring water is the purest choice, while herbs such as chamomile or green tea will provide more subtle benefits. Hot water extracts more starch, making the rice water thicker, while cold water gives it a softer feel.

Find your balance:

This is where the magic begins.
The classic 1::1 ratio (1 cup rice: 1 cup water) is a good starting point. But your skin, like the skin of a savvy music lover, has its own preferences.
Drier skin types may need a 1::2 ratio to replenish moisture,
while oily skin types may prefer a 1::1.5 ratio for a lighter feel.

Remember that beauty is a personal symphony: **Start light:** Start with dilution and gradually increase concentration as your skin adapts. Don't rush to reach the top! Listen to your skin: Pay attention to any signs of irritation or discomfort.
Each skin is a unique tool, so adjust the proportions accordingly.

Experiment with variations: Explore different types of rice, water temperatures, and even add a little honey or aloe vera for added benefits. Each note adds depth to your symphony of beauty. **Beyond formula:**
Nourish from within: Remember that true beauty radiates from within.
Eat a healthy diet, manage stress, and prioritize sleep for a healthy foundation. Think of it like tuning your instrument before any performance.

Seek professional advice: If you have a pre-existing skin condition, consult a dermatologist before incorporating rice water into your routine. Let the experts harmonise your skin care symphony. Embrace the journey:

Enjoy the process of discovering natural ingredients and creating your own unique beauty rituals. Remember, the most radiant beauty comes from self-discovery and love for your unique skin. So, put aside your worries and enter the bustling rice market.
With a little experimentation and a mindful approach, you will create a rice water formula that meets your skin's unique needs, leaving you radiant and beautiful, in perfect harmony. Remember, the most captivating music is often the music that touches your unique soul.

3 Waltz of the rice fields: Soaking time and temperature - To suit your beauty tone Rice water, the new beauty muse, invites you with the promise of radiant skin . But amid rumours about the soaking method, confusion still reigns.

Fear not, beauty detective! Today we dive into the fascinating world of soaking times and temperatures, helping you tailor the tone of your rice water to your skin's unique rhythms.

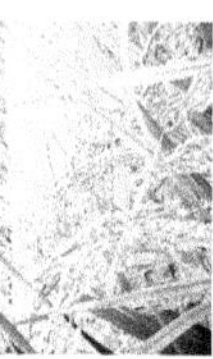

This image: a rice field bathed in sunlight, each grain of rice swaying gently in the wind. Water, reflecting the heat of the sun, has the potential to be a beauty elixir. But just as a waltz requires the right tempo and steps, so does your journey through rice water.

A Symphony of Soaking Time: A Soothing Music (30 Minutes): Perfect for sensitive skin, a 30-minute soak will release a gentle tone of nutrients, providing moisture. Lightly moisturising and soothing feeling. Think of it as a subtle prelude that gently awakens your skin.

A Flourishing Aria (1-2 hours):
For normal to dry skin, an extended soak of up to 1-2 hours will deepen the tone, extracting more starches for a richer experience. richer, more nutritious. Think of it as a boost of hydration, leaving your skin plump and dewy.

A Power Ride (Night): For those seeking a truly transformative experience, an overnight soak will unleash a full symphony of nutrients.
Think of it as a grand finale, revealing rice's deepest secrets for a powerful beauty boost.
But remember that this trip may not be suitable for all skin types, so approach it with caution.

Warm hug: Cool hug: Cold water whispers a refreshing melody, ideal for oily or acne-prone skin. It tightens pores and minimise sebum production, leaving your skin feeling invigorated and balanced.

Warm Resonance: Warm water provides a soothing sensation, perfect for normal or sensitive skin. It promotes gentle nutrient extraction while remaining gentle on your skin.

Hot Spring Serenade: Hot Water sings a rich melody, ideal for dry skin. It releases the most starch, creating a thicker rice water for intense hydration.

But keep in mind that this hot spring may be too strong for sensitive skin, so be careful. Remember that beauty is a personal component:

Start with a gentle tone: Start with shorter soak times and cooler temperatures, gradually increasing as your skin adapts. Don't rush the pace! Listen to your skin: Pay attention to any signs of irritation or discomfort.

Each skin is a separate instrument, so adjust the soaking time and temperature accordingly. **Experiment with variations:** Explore different combinations of soaking times and temperatures to find the right one for your skin. Each note adds depth to your symphony of beauty. Beyond formula:

Nourish from within: Remember that true beauty radiates from within. Eat a healthy diet, manage stress, and prioritise sleep for a healthy foundation. Think of it like tuning your instrument before any performance.

Seek professional advice: If you have a pre-existing skin condition, consult a dermatologist before incorporating rice water into your routine. Let the experts harmonise your skin care symphony.

Embrace the journey: Enjoy the process of discovering natural ingredients and creating your own unique beauty rituals. Remember, the most radiant beauty comes from self-discovery and love for your unique skin as you step into the sunny rice fields on your beauty journey.

With a mindful approach and a little experimentation, you'll discover the perfect soaking time and temperature to create the rice water tone that leaves your skin radiant and beautiful, in perfect harmony with the rhythm. its own uniqueness. Remember, the most captivating music is often the music that touches your unique soul.

Chapter 5

Cauldron of Fire: Unleash the power of boiled rice water Rice water, the new muse of beauty, beckons with the promise of radiant skin. But for those looking for a stronger, more potent elixir, the boiling method has some potential. Imagine a cauldron of fire turning humble grains of rice into a rich, nutrient-rich brew, ready to work its magic on your skin. But remember that the exercise of this power comes with responsibility!

The Secret of the Cauldron: The Symphony of Starches: Unlike the sweet melodies of soaking, boiling produces a powerful release of starch. This creates a thicker, more viscous rice water, ideal for dry or mature skin looking for deep hydration and plumping. Think of it as a rich sauce, nourishing your skin with concentrated nutrients.

Fast and fiery: No time for a slow waltz? The boiling method allows for quick processing. In just 15 minutes, your powerful elixir will be ready. Think of it like a fiery dance, releasing the rice grain's hidden treasures in a blast of heat.

A balancing act: with great power comes responsibility. The effectiveness of rice water may not be suitable for all skin types. Sensitive skin may feel too harsh, so err on the side of caution and prioritise patch testing.

Recipe Revealed: Gather Ingredients: 1/2 cup uncooked rice (brown or white), 2 cups water, a saucepan, and a fine mesh strainer. Think of them as the tools you need to create your beauty potion.
Light a fire: Boil water, the pot boils like a miniature volcano. Next, add the rice as if you were offering grain to the fire god.

Fiery Dance: Soak rice in boiling water for 15 minutes, to release its secrets in a fiery dance. **Cooling:** Once the dance is complete, strain your fiery elixir into a clean container, allowing it to cool before using. Think of it as a stabilising medicine, its power waiting to be harnessed in that beauty is a personal concoction: Start with a diluted potion:

Even the most powerful mages do not start at their full power. Start by diluting the rice water with cold water to avoid irritation. Listen to your skin: Pay attention to how your skin reacts. If you feel discomfort, switch to gentler methods or seek professional advice.

Experiment with variations: Explore by adding a little honey for a soothing effect or essential oils for a personal fragrance. Each ingredient adds a unique touch to your beauty routine.

Beyond the Cauldron: Nourish from within: Remember that true beauty radiates from the inside out. Eat a healthy diet, manage stress, and prioritise sleep for a healthy foundation. Think of this as building a sturdy cauldron before brewing your potion.
Seek expert advice: If you have a pre-existing skin condition, consult a dermatologist before incorporating boiled rice water into your routine. Let the experts guide you in using this powerful ingredient safely.
Embrace the journey: Enjoy the process of discovering natural ingredients and creating your own unique beauty rituals. Remember, the most radiant beauty comes from self-discovery and love for your unique skin as you play the role of beauty alchemist and embrace the fiery cauldron of the boiling method.
With a mindful approach and a little caution, you can unlock the secrets of this powerful elixir, leaving your skin nourished and radiant. Remember that the most powerful spells are performed with respect and understanding of your own needs.

1 Step-by-step instruction and safety precautions.

In this guide, we'll explore boiling, a technique that produces a richer extract. Follow these steps with visuals to improve your understanding and ensure safety precautions are in place.

Step 1: Collect ingredients - Collect the necessary ingredients, including plants, water, pots and heat sources.

Step 2: Prepare the plant - Clean and cut the plant to desired size for extraction. Make sure they are fresh and high quality for best results.

Step 3: Boil water - Pour water into a pot and boil over heat source. Use enough water to cover the plant being extracted.

Step 4: Add plants - Once the water boils, carefully add the prepared plants to the pot. Stir gently to ensure even extraction.

Step 5: Simmer - Reduce heat to boiling and let herbs soak in water. Monitor the process to avoid overflow.

Step 6: Extract the rich flavour - Boil the plant for the recommended time to extract the rich flavour. Stir occasionally for even extraction.

Step 7: Filter the extract - Once the extraction process is complete, filter the extract to separate the liquid from the plant. Use a fine mesh strainer or cheesecloth for this step.

Step 8: Store and enjoy - Transfer the extract into a clean jar and store properly.

Enjoy your rich extract in various culinary or medicinal applications.

Safety precautions: - Use caution when handling hot water and steam during boiling. - Keep a safe distance from heat sources to avoid accidents. - Use appropriate cooking utensils and equipment to avoid burns or injuries

By following the step-by-step instructions and safety precautions, you can master the boiling method to create a richer extract.

Experiment with different plants and enjoy the flavorful results of your extraction.

2.Unlock flavour (and nutrients!): Optimise your boiling ritual Boiling, often thought of as a cooking tool, can be more than just a way to heat water . With a few tweaks and tricks, you can turn it into a powerful tool for extracting maximum flavour and nutrients from your ingredients.

1: Know your enemies (and your allies): Heat is the villain: High temperatures can break down vitamins and minerals. Aim for a gentle boil (think happy little bubbles) rather than a hard boil.

Water is your double agent: It filters nutrients and carries them into your broth. Use the minimum amount of water, just enough to cover your ingredients as you can always add more later if needed.

Step 2: Harness the power of acids: A little vinegar, lemon juice or even yogurt can work wonders. Acidity helps break down cell walls, making nutrients more accessible.

Reward: it will add brightness to your broth!

Step 3: Discover the magic of aromatics: Don't throw away your ingredients – infuse them! Add whole herbs, spices, garlic, ginger or even onion skins for added flavour and health benefits. Think of it as a simmering spice for your broth.

Step 4: Make friends with fats: A drop of olive oil or coconut oil can help retain fat-soluble vitamins like A, D and E, preventing them from escaping with steam. Plus, it gives your broth a silky feel.

Step 5: Time Travel Precautions: Overcooking is a nutrient thief! Respect the minimum cooking time required for your ingredients to soften. Remember that some nutrients are more sensitive to heat than others.

For example, green leafy vegetables only need to be soaked quickly. Safety first! Never boil without supervision. Use a pot with a tight-fitting lid to minimise nutrient loss through steam. Be aware of potential allergens in the herbs and flavourings you choose.

Bonus tip : Don't throw away nutrient-rich broth! Use it in soups, stews, sauces or even rice to add flavour and a health boost to your entire meal. Remember that boiling is a journey, not a destination.

Experiment, have fun and discover the hidden potential of this simple yet powerful technique. With a little knowledge and creativity, you can transform your boiling game and unlock a world of rich, delicious, nutrient-dense dishes!

3 The dance of proportions: Finding the right balance between flavour and function Imagine your kitchen as a laboratory, ingredients as your dance partners and proportions is choreography.

Choosing the right ratio for the desired concentration is like creating the perfect performance: a delicate balance between expression and precision. But don't worry, dear culinary alchemist! Don't be afraid of the cup, because with just a little understanding and a little creativity, you will quickly become a master theorist.

1. Know your players: Solute: The star of the show, the flavour you want to focus on. Coffee grounds, herbs, and spices all play this role. Solvent: Your carrier, flavour carrier. Water, broth, oil, all are waiting in the chicken wings.

2. Understanding Desire: Intensity: Do you crave a bold, stand-out punch or a subtle whisper of flavour? Adjust your rates accordingly. Texture: Velvety soft, or a symphony of textures?

Different ratios may affect the final consistency.

3. Tango Ratio: Start with a Baseline: Find the general ratio for the solute and solvent you have chosen. This is your starting point, not your final action. Adjust and taste: Don't be afraid to experiment! Start with a small batch and gradually adjust the proportions, tasting as you go. Remember, the palace is your ultimate guide.

Think beyond the numbers: Consider the other ingredients in your recipe. Are there any natural flavour enhancers or reducers? Adjust your rates accordingly.

Professional tips for perfect performance: **Temperature issues**: Heat can affect the extraction process. Experiment with boiling, brewing or even cold brewing to find your sweetness.

Time is of the essence: Over-extraction can lead to a bitter taste. Respect the time needed to get maximum flavour without sacrificing quality. Respect for ingredients: Fresh, high-quality ingredients taste better and deliver more vibrant flavours.

Don't be The perfect ratio is a personal journey. Don't be afraid to break the mould, experiment and above all have fun! With each successful performance, you will become a master of concentration, opening the door to a world of culinary possibilities. Now go ahead and create your masterpiece!

Chapter 6

Fermentation fest: Where bacteria meet flavour! Ditch the pressure cooker, ditch the blender – fermentation is the secret weapon in your culinary arsenal, waiting to unleash a symphony of flavours and health benefits. It's not just frothy kimchi and tangy yoghourt; It's a lively party where microscopic friends turn simple ingredients into flavour bombs and nutritional powerhouses.

Buckle up because we're about to get into a wild carnival! The magic of bacteria: Imagine tiny, invisible chefs working tirelessly in your kitchen, breaking down sugar and creating a kaleidoscope of flavours and nutrients. This is the magic of fermentation!

These friendly microbes, like bacteria and yeast, unleash the hidden potential of your ingredients, giving you: Intense Flavour: Imagine deeper, richer flavours of vegetables, brighter flavours of fruit, and bursts of umami in everything from soy sauce to miso.

Nutritional Enhancement: fermentation increases the bioavailability of vitamins and minerals, making them easier for your body to absorb. Consider gut-friendly probiotics, vitamin K2 and even B vitamins.

Preservability: By creating an acidic environment, fermentation extends the shelf life of foods naturally, reducing waste and allowing you to 'save money'. Fiesta Fermentation Menu: The possibilities are endless!

Here are some ideas to whet your taste buds: Vegetable Festival:

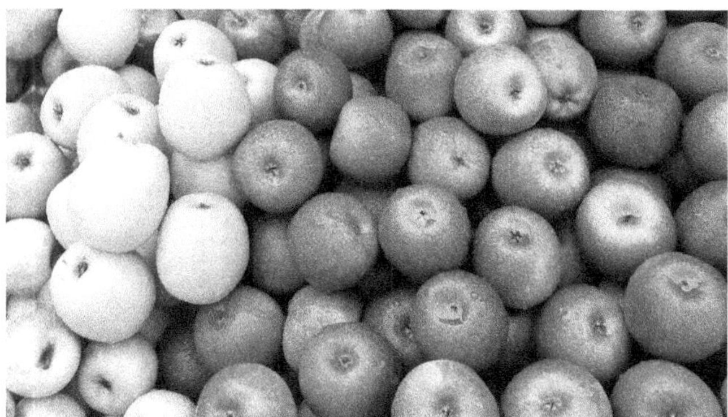

Sauerkraut, kimchi, marinated peppers, curtido – the crunchy and aromatic world of fermented vegetables awaits you!

Dairy goodness: Yoghourt, kefir, buttermilk - creamy, probiotic goodness for breakfast, snacks or even dips.

Cheap drinks: Kombucha, kefir water, tepache – delicious, fizzy drinks that quench your thirst and nourish your gut. Breads and more: Sourdough bread, idli, dosa – staples that are moist, flavorful and packed with nutrition.

Are you ready to join the party? Fermentation is surprisingly easy and accessible. All you need are basic ingredients, a little patience, and a willingness to experiment.

There are countless resources online and in libraries to guide you on your journey which it's not about perfection but about discovering and enjoying the wonderful fruits of your microbial collaboration. So what are you waiting for?

Grab your ingredients, release the bacteria, and get ready to experience the magic of fermentation! It's a delicious, healthy, and endlessly creative adventure waiting for you to enjoy.

1. A step-by-step guide to fermentation: Decoding the magic of bacteria Embark on a fascinating journey into the world of fermentation, where bacteria work their magic to turn ordinary ingredients into extraordinary creations.

Let's dive into the step-by-step process and reveal the principles behind this ancient alchemy.

1: Choose ingredients - Start by choosing fresh, high-quality ingredients for fermentation. Choose your base ingredients, such as vegetables, fruits or grains, along with any additional flavourings.

Step 2: Prepare the fermentation tank - Clean and disinfect the fermentation tank to create a favourable environment for beneficial bacteria. Make sure it is free of any contaminants.

Step 3: Mix ingredients - Mix selected ingredients in the fermentation tank, making sure they are evenly distributed. Add spices or seasonings to enhance the flavour.

Step 4: Add starter culture - Add starter culture or a product containing beneficial bacteria to restart the fermentation process. This culture will begin the process of converting sugar into acids and gases.

Step 5: Sealing and preservation - Cover the fermentation vessel with a tight lid or fermentation lock to create an ideal anaerobic environment for microbial activity. Place the container in a dark place and at room temperature.

Step 6: Watch and wait - Monitor the fermentation process, observing changes in color, texture and aroma. Give bacteria time to work their magic, transforming ingredients into a delicious product.

Step 7: Taste and testing - After the fermentation period, taste a small sample of the fermented product to evaluate the flavour and readiness of the product. Adjust seasoning or fermentation time if necessary.

Fermentation principles: - Microbial diversity: Different bacterial strains contribute to unique flavours and textures during fermentation.

Adjust pH: Bacteria produce acids that have the function of adjusting the pH of the fermentation environment, preserving the product and enhancing flavour.

Anaerobic conditions: Fermentation occurs in the absence of oxygen, creating a favourable environment for beneficial microorganisms to grow. - Time and temperature: Fermentation rate changes with temperature and time, affecting the characteristics of the final product.

Master the art of fermentation with step-by-step instructions enriched and guided by the principles of microbial alchemy. Witness the transformative power of bacteria, creating delicious yeasts that delight the taste buds and nourish the body.

2. Embark on a Fermentation Journey: The Dance of Vigilance and Conservation As you delve into the exciting realm of fermentation, mastering the art of monitoring progress and protecting against spoilage is The simple thing.

Let's explore a unique approach to vigilance and conservation during fermentation, ensuring your creativity flourishes and delights the senses. The dance of tracking fermentation progress:

Step 1: Visual inspection - Engage your senses in a visual feast as you observe the changes occurring in the fermentation tank . Look for bubbles, colour changes and texture variations as signs of active fermentation.

Step 2: Fragrance in the air - Breathe in the enchanting aromas emanating from the fermentation tank, a symphony of microbial activity. Note any unpleasant odours that may indicate deterioration and intervene promptly.

Step 3: Taste Test - Treat yourself to the ritual of tasting a small sample of the yeast to gauge its flavour development. Trust your taste to detect the nuances and adjust fermentation time or seasoning accordingly. The art of avoiding spoilage:

Step 1: Maintaining sanitary conditions - Maintain a clean and hygienic environment throughout the fermentation process to prevent harmful contaminants from affecting your work.

Step 2: Seal and store properly - Seal the fermentation tank securely to create an anaerobic environment conducive to the growth of beneficial microorganisms. Store the container in a cool, dark place, away from direct sunlight.

Step 3: Control pH and temperature - Monitor the pH levels of the fermentation to ensure they remain within the optimal range for microbial activity. Maintain a stable temperature to aid fermentation.

Step 4: Trust your instincts - Cultivate a sense of intuition when detecting signs of deterioration. When in doubt, err on the side of caution and discard any ferments with unusual properties. The Dance of Vigilance and Conservation Fermentation is a harmonious combination of initiative and awakening of the senses

In the symphony of dilution and preservation, balance and rest blend together to create a harmonious melody that takes your fermentation to new heights. By following these unique instructions and suggestions, you will foster a deep connection with your creations and nurture them to their full potential, creating a symphony of flavor. Taste satisfies the senses and nourishes the soul.

Chapter 7

Unleash the magic of soaked rice: Elevate the elixir beyond the ordinary. Immerse yourself in a world where ordinary rice is transformed into a picture of creativity and happiness. Discover the art of making rice water that goes beyond the usual elixirs, infused with a touch of magic and a dash of ingenuity. Let's go beyond the basics and discover the secrets of making rice water that captivates the senses and nourishes the spirit.

Infusion Alchemy:
Step 1: Botanical Bliss - Immerse yourself in rice water in a botanical symphony of herbs, flowers and spices. Let the essence of nature infuse your elixir with vibrant flavours and healing benefits.

Step 2: Citrus Zest - Enhance the flavour of your latte with a touch of citrus peel, adding a refreshing and invigorating kick to your rice water. Apply bright and lively notes to awaken the senses.

Step 3: Aromatic Adventure - Embark on an aromatic journey with exotic spices and aromatics. Let the warmth of cinnamon, the earthiness of cardamom or the floral notes of lavender weave a flavour into your rice water.

Symphony of Creation:

Step 1: Mindful Preparation - Approach the creation of rice soak with mindfulness and intention. Let each ingredient reflect your creativity and be a source of nourishment for body and mind.

Step 2: Infusion Ritual - Participate in the infusion ritual, letting the flavours blend and develop over time. Embrace the transformative power of patience as your rice water elixir matures and grows in complexity.

Step 3: Enjoy Elixir - Enjoy the sensory experience of enjoying your soaked rice water product. May each sip be a moment of mindfulness, a celebration of flavour and a journey to discover the depth of flavour.

Beyond the basics are endless possibilities, where rice water recipes become a playground for creativity and a sanctuary for self-care. Capture the magic of infusions, take your elixir to the next level and let the alchemy of flavours and aromas transport you to a culinary world of enchantment and bliss.

1 Embrace the bounty of nature: A symphony of herbs, flowers and natural alchemy In the tapestry of culinary creativity, herbs, flowers and Other natural ingredients appear in brilliant strokes that paint a masterpiece of flavour and essence. .
Embark on a journey through the garden of possibilities, where the richness of nature blends with the art of mixology and culinary alchemy. Discover the magic of adding herbs, flowers and other natural ingredients to take your creations to new heights of well-being and holistic nutrition.

The Herbal Ensemble:

Step 1: Herbaceous Harmony - Harness the aromatic power of herbs like basil, rosemary and thyme to create a symphony of flavour in your dishes. Let the herbs dance on your palate, creating a fresh and deep tone.

Step 2: Healing Elixirs - Discover the healing properties of herbs like chamomile, mint and lavender, turning your creations into healing elixirs that soothe the body and calm the mind. Enjoy the comprehensive benefits of natural medicine.

Step 3: Culinary Creativity - Awaken your inner alchemist by experimenting with oils, vinegars and herb-based syrups. Let the versatility of herbs inspire your culinary creativity and elevate simple dishes into culinary masterpieces.

Floral Symphony:

Step 1: Petal Poetry - Infuse your creations with the delicate beauty and fragrance of edible flowers such as roses, violets and hibiscus. Let the poetry of flower petals spread across your plate, adding elegance and magic to your dish.

2: Floral Infusions - Immerse yourself in a world of floral scents, where floral essences such as jasmine, elderflower and orange blossom transform drinks and desserts into fragrant works of art. Let the floral symphony mesmerize your senses.

Step 3: Kitchen Aromatherapy - Immerse yourself in the world of kitchen aromatherapy, where floral scents awaken memories, lift spirits and enhance the dining experience. Let the fragrance of flowers transport you to a realm of blissful feelings.

In the garden of culinary creativity, herbs, flowers and natural ingredients flourish as essential tools to prepare dishes that nourish the body, stimulate the taste buds and elevate the soul. Immerse yourself in the symphony of nature's bounty, imbue your creativity with the magic of herbs and flowers, and let the alchemy of natural ingredients guide you on your journey. culinary exploration and sensory pleasure.

2 Skin Alchemy: Create elixirs to transform dry and oily skin In the realm of skin care alchemy, formulas tailored to specific concerns skin becomes a transformative medicine, combining botanical wonders and natural remedies to solve skin problems.
Special needs of oily and dry skin. Join me on a journey through the magical garden of skincare, where the power of nature and the art of preparation converge to create elixirs that heal, balance and rejuvenate the skin.

Join us to discover the secret to creating formulas for dry and oily skin, harnessing the wisdom of herbs, oils and essences to deliver radiance and vitality.

For oily skin:

Step 1: Balancing Act - Leverages the balancing properties of ingredients like witch hazel, tea tree oil and green tea to regulate sebum production and purify skin. Let these botanical allies restore harmony to oily skin and reveal clear, smooth skin.

Step 2: Clarifying concoction - Use clarifying herbs like thyme, rosemary and neem in your recipes to fight acne, reduce inflammation and shrink pores. Let the purifying essence of these botanical wonders cleanse and revitalise oily skin.

Step 3: Hydration Harmony - Find the balance between hydration and oil control by incorporating lightweight yet nourishing oils like jojoba, grapeseed and argan into your skin care formula. Let these moisturisers quench your skin's thirst without clogging pores, leaving your skin soft, smooth and glowing.

For dry skin:

Step 1: Moisture Magic - Wraps your skin in a cocoon of moisture with ingredients like hyaluronic acid, shea butter and avocado oil to replenish nutrients. dry and dehydrated skin. Let these moisturising emollients restore elasticity, softness and vitality to parched skin.

Step 2: Soothing Serum - Soothes and nourishes dry, sensitive skin with skin-soothing botanicals such as chamomile, chamomile and oat extracts. Let the gentle touch of these botanicals reduce redness, irritation and discomfort, restoring peace to the skin barrier.

Step 3: Radiance Revival - Brightens dry skin with antioxidant and vitamin-rich ingredients like rosehip seed oil, vitamin E and aloe vera. Let these rejuvenating elixirs boost collagen production, fade dark spots and give skin a healthy glow, revealing skin that radiates beauty from the inside out.

In the Alchemical Skin Care Formula Lab, formulas for oily and dry skin problems become transformative rituals of self-care and rejuvenation. Harness the power of natural remedies, infuse your skin care creations with intention and mindfulness, and let the alchemy of botanical ingredients guide you on the path to Radiant, balanced and healthy skin.

Part 3

Revealing the Asian gem: The ritual of drinking rice water for radiant skin Rice water, the elixir of Asian beauty secrets, is no longer just for nourishing grains. Its journey has gone beyond the kitchen and onto bathroom shelves as a powerful natural skin care product. But forget boring, starchy recipes: we're about to embark on a rice water transformation ritual!

Step 1: The journey to find the perfect pearl: Choose your rice wisely: Choose unpolished rice varieties like brown or jasmine because they retain more nutrients.
Organic is always a plus! Water Dance: Experiment! Soaking in filtered water releases vitamins and minerals, while fermentation creates a powerful probiotic blend. Choose your method based on your skin's needs.

Step 2: Cooking rice water: Soaking method: Cleaning process: Wash rice thoroughly to remove impurities. Sweet Sleep: Soak rice in filtered water for 1 to 2 hours or overnight for stronger fermentation. Filter the essence: Filter the rice water through cheesecloth, separating the liquid gold from the grains.

Fermentation method: The Bubbly Wake Up: Soak the rice in filtered water for 1-2 days, so that the rice begins to naturally ferment. (Caution: This method may have a stronger smell.) Strain the elixir: Strain the fermented rice water, removing any remaining solids.

Step 3: Infuses the power of rice into skin: Cleanses skin: Gently massage cold rice water onto face and neck, using it as a natural facial cleanser or makeup remover.
The Toning Touch: Dip a cotton pad in rice water and apply to skin for a refreshing, pH-balanced toner.

The Mystical Mask: Combine rice water with other skin-loving ingredients like honey or aloe vera to create a skin-nourishing mask. Leave for 15 to 20 minutes and rinse with warm water. **Remember**: Consistency is key! Use rice water regularly to see its full benefits. However, listen to your skin and adjust frequency or method as needed.

Bonus tip : Don't throw away leftover rice! Cook it as usual, knowing that its nutrients have been partially extracted from your beauty potion.

Embark on this rice water ritual and witness the transformation of your skin. From a gentle cleanser to a brightening mask, this ancient wisdom holds the key to radiant, healthy skin. So, drop the Asian gem into your kitchen and let your skin benefit from its transformative power!

Chapter 8

Dawn Before Dazzle: Lay the foundation for a flawless foundation with cleansing and toning Imagine your skin as a masterpiece waiting to be revealed. But before decorating with vibrant colours and intricate details, an important step **lays the foundation**: cleaning and staining . Think of it as the sunrise before the dazzle, preparing your painting for you a radiant transformation.

The Cleaning Caper: Unmasking Impurities: Imagine your cleanser as a gentle detective, removing makeup, dirt and pollutants like tiny clues to a mystery . Choose your weapons wisely: creams for dry skin, lightweight gels for oily skin and Micellar water for total refreshment.

Remember to be gentle: vigorous rubbing is the enemy! Balance: Imagine your skin's pH as the pH of a tightrope walker. Cleaning can disrupt this balance, but don't worry! Choose a cleanser with a balanced pH to maintain natural harmony, giving you fresh and comfortable skin.

Firming Symphony: Restore Harmony: Think of toner as a conductor, regulating the pH of your skin after cleansing. Choose an alcohol-free formula with gentle ingredients like rose water or witch hazel for dry skin or green tea for oily skin. Swipe it onto your face and feel the cool embrace that restores balance.

The finishing touch: Think of ink as the final stroke, preparing your canvas for the next stage. It removes any remaining impurities and ensures your serums and moisturisers can work their magic more effectively.

Beyond the basics: Customization conundrums: Remember, one size does not fit all! Experiment with different cleansers and toners to find the perfect one for your skin type and concerns.

The Consistency Cadence: Cleansing and toning your skin are not one-time events. Make them a daily routine, morning and evening, to maintain a healthy and balanced foundation.

The Gentle Touch: Always be gentle with your skin! Avoid rubbing and tugging and use circular motions for optimal cleaning. Remember: Cleansing and toning are the first steps in your skin care journey.

Applying this firm foundation will leave your skin truly glowing, ready to embrace the vibrant colours and textures in your personal skincare routine. So go ahead, cleanse, tone and unleash your skin's masterpiece!

1.The Rice Renaissance:

Turn grains into glowing skin Forget harsh chemicals and fancy cleansers, your skin craves a little Oriental flavour! Rice water, the ancient Asian beauty elixir, is no longer just used to nourish grains.

It's about to become the secret weapon in your cleansing and toning arsenal, offering a gentle yet effective approach to glowing skin. But before you get started, let's explore the techniques that will allow you to exploit its full potential.

Cleansing Waterfall: Perform a Geisha Ritual: Tune into your inner geisha by using rice water as a gentle cleanser. Dip a cotton pad in cooked rice water and apply it to your face to remove makeup and impurities. Think of it as a gentle caress, leaving your skin feeling fresh and clean.

The Double Cleanse Dance: For a deep clean, combine rice water with a gentle, natural cleanser. Massage the mixture onto your face, letting the soothing properties of the rice water work their magic while the cleanser draws away stubborn impurities. Rinse off and enjoy the balanced, soft feeling.

Micellar Magic: if you are a Micellar water lover, try mixing it with rice water! Mix in equal parts and soak a cotton pad. Gently apply to face to take advantage of the dual cleansing power of micelles and the brightening properties of rice water.

The Toning Touch: The Surprising Spritz: Brings the refreshing feeling of rice water mist. Fill a spray bottle with cold rice water and lightly spray it on your face after washing your face. This energises the skin, balances pH levels and prepares the skin for serum or moisturiser.

The Calm Compress: For a soothing sensation, soak a washcloth in cool rice water and gently apply to your face. Keep it on for a few minutes to let the soothing properties of rice water work its magic, reducing redness and inflammation.

The Mystical Mask: Treat your skin with a rice water facial mask. Mix rice water with other skin-loving ingredients like honey or aloe vera. Apply the mask generously and leave it on for 15 to 20 minutes. Rinse with warm water and enjoy plump, hydrated skin.

Remember: Don't just clean and tone, transform! Imagine rice water gently removing impurities, leaving your skin as smooth and receptive as a newly polished pearl. Imagine nutrients being restored to balance, like a gentle wave lapping on a sunny beach.

Perform the ritual: Persistence is the key: Cleansing and toning your skin regularly with rice water will unleash its full potential. However, listen to your skin and adjust frequency or method as needed.

Bonus tip : Don't throw away leftover rice! Cook it as usual, knowing that its nutrients have been partially extracted from your beauty potion.

As you enter the world of rice water, where ancient wisdom meets modern beauty routines. Unleash this gem in your kitchen and let your skin benefit from its transformative power! Remember that the rice renaissance has begun and invite you to join the radiant revolution!

2.The Dance of the Skin: Balances pH for Radiant Harmony Imagine your skin as a vibrant ecosystem, teeming with microscopic life and bubbling with activity. At the heart of this ecosystem is a vital element:

pH balance . It is the invisible conductor that coordinates the harmony of the skin's natural defence system and keeps it healthy and radiant. But what happens when this delicate dance is interrupted?

Nasty culprits: Harsh cleansers: Think of them as bulldozers, stripping away your skin's natural oils and disrupting the delicate pH balance. This leaves your skin tight, dry and vulnerable.

Environmental stressors: Pollution, sun exposure and even hard water can act as mischievous agents, disrupting your skin's pH. This can lead to irritation, redness, and even premature aging.

Food Choices: What goes in affects what comes out! Sugary and processed foods can create an acidic environment internally, which can affect the skin's pH, leading to acne and dull skin. **Restoring harmony:** Fear not, flesh adventurer! There are many ways to be your skin's pH leader and bring about a harmonious dance:

Gentle cleansers: Choose a pH-balanced cleanser that works like the doers gently garden, removes impurities without affecting the natural balance. Consider cream formulas containing hyaluronic acid or ceramides to keep your skin hydrated and youthful.

Toning Tales: pH-balancing toner can act like a gentle balm, restoring the skin's natural acidity after cleansing. Choose alcohol-free formulas with soothing ingredients like rose water or witch hazel to gently rebalance your skin's ecosystem.

Dietary Dance: Nourish your skin from the inside out by incorporating fruits, vegetables and healthy fats into your diet. Think of them as vitamins for your skin, helping to maintain a healthy internal pH, reflecting your external glow.

Consistency is key! Regular use of pH-balancing products and maintaining a healthy lifestyle will help your skin maintain optimal pH and achieve radiant, healthy skin.

Beyond the basics: Listen to your skin: Pay attention to its signals. If you experience dryness, irritation, or breakouts, this could be a sign of disturbed pH. Adjust your routine and consider consulting a dermatologist if necessary.

Prebiotics and Probiotics: Consider combining prebiotic and probiotic skin care products or supplements. These can help support the good bacteria on your skin, contributing to a healthy microbiome and pH balance.

Embrace the journey: Think of balancing your pH not as a chore but as a fascinating journey of discovery. With a little knowledge and the right tools, you can unlock the secrets of your skin's ecosystem and watch it dance with newfound joy. So go ahead, become the leader of skin harmony and experience the radiant skin that awaits you!

Chapter 9

Beyond the Basics: Masquerade Ball - Unleash Your Skin's Inner Alchemist Forget the same old skin care routine, your skin craves adventure! Masks and treatments are the secret weapons in your beauty arsenal, waiting to unleash a world of personalised transformations. Abandon autopilot and embark on a journey to discover your skin's hidden potential, one mask at a time.

Unmasking the magic: Imagine yourself at a masked ball, each mask representing a different aspect of your desired skin: Le Havre Moisturizer: You Does it feel dry and tight? Enjoy the plumping power of a hydrating mask.

Consider hyaluronic acid, aloe vera, or even homemade options like avocado and honey. Imagine your skin quenching its thirst, becoming soft and supple, like a happy guest enjoying a refreshing drink.
The Detox Dance: Does city life bore you? Unleash the purifying power of a clay or charcoal mask. Imagine them drawing out impurities like tiny magnets, leaving your skin feeling refreshed and energised, like a dancer shedding her heavy costume after a powerful performance.

Goddess of Light: Do you want to light up the light within you? Look no further than skin-brightening face masks made with vitamin C, turmeric, or even lemon juice.

Imagine your skin bathed in radiant light, ready to conquer the day, like a spotlight finding its perfect star. Anti-Aging Alchemy: Time stands no chance against the powerful ingredients in anti-aging masks.

Think peptides, retinol and antioxidants that work wonders in fighting wrinkles. Imagine your skin defying gravity, regaining youthful elasticity, like a magician reversing time with a simple wave of his wand. Beyond the Mask: The mask is just the beginning!

Explore the world of targeted care: Serums: These concentrated elixirs deliver powerful doses of actives like niacinamide for imperfections or hyaluronic acid for hydration. Think of them as personalised potions, each with its own charm to enhance the beauty of your skin.

Exfoliation: Gentle exfoliation or chemical peels will remove dead skin cells, resulting in brighter, smoother skin. Imagine them removing dullness like an experienced painter removing layers to reveal a vibrant masterpiece.

Facial Oil: These nourishing blends lock in moisture and deliver essential fatty acids. Think of them as luxurious treatments that leave your skin feeling soft and supple, like a queen receiving an aromatic massage. Make masks and treatments a regular part of your routine, but listen to your skin. Adjust frequency and type based on your personal needs and climate.

Bonus tip : Don't forget your neck and chest! These areas often show signs of ageing first, so extend your treatment to them. So, step away from the mundane and embrace the transformative power of masks and treatments.

With a little experimentation and the right tools, you can unleash your skin's inner alchemist and witness its breathtaking transformation. Remember, your skin is a canvas waiting to be adorned with vibrant health and beauty. Go ahead, create your masterpiece and let the charades begin!

1.From Attic to Shine: Make a Magical Rice Water Face Mask Ditch the store-bought potions and tap into ancient wisdom (and your pantry!) with face mask recipes. Rice water is simple and effective.

Imagine your skin enjoying the gentle yet powerful power of rice water, leaving it radiant and vibrant. So roll up your sleeves and unleash your inner kitchen alchemist! The

Hydrating Haven: Honeycomb Bliss: Mash a ripe banana with a teaspoon of honey and mix with 1/4 cup of rice water.
This cream mixture contains lots of moisture and antioxidants, making your skin soft and supple like a baby's skin. Apply and leave for 15 minutes before rinsing.

Cool Cucumber: Mix cucumber with 1/2 cup of rice water to create a cooling and hydrating mask. The cooling properties of cucumber will soothe irritated skin, while rice water provides a boost of vitamins and minerals.

Apply and relax for 15 to 20 minutes before rinsing. The Detox Dance: Clay Caper: Mix 1 tablespoon green clay with 1/4 cup rice water and a few drops of tea tree oil. This powerful mask will remove impurities and excess oil, leaving your skin clean and refreshed.

Apply and let dry before rinsing gently with warm water. Oasis Oats: Mix 1 tablespoon ground oatmeal with 1/3 cup rice water and a little honey.
This gentle mask exfoliates and absorbs excess oil, leaving your skin relaxed and balanced. Apply and massage gently before rinsing with warm water.

Shining Goddess: Twisted Turmeric: Mix 1 tablespoon natural yogurt with 1/4 cup rice water and a pinch of turmeric powder. This brightening mask will even out your skin tone and give you a radiant glow. Apply and leave for 10 to 15 minutes before rinsing with warm water.

Rosewater Radiance: Mix 1/4 cup of rice water with 2 tablespoons of rose water and a few drops of lemon juice. This refreshing mask will revitalise your skin and make it look brighter.

Apply and leave for 10 minutes before rinsing with warm water. Additional tips: Don't throw away leftover rice water! Use it as a toner or face mist to enjoy its benefits throughout the day.

Consistency is key! Use these masks regularly for optimal results. However, listen to your skin and adjust ingredients or frequency of use if necessary. So, ditch the complicated habits and embrace the simple magic of rice water.

With a little creativity and these easy recipes, you can achieve radiant, healthy skin that reflects your unique beauty. Remember, light starts in your kitchen, so grab your whisk and let the rice water transformation begin!

2.The Rice Water Revolution: Infuse your skin care routine with ancient wisdom Forget the endless product line, your skin craves a little Oriental flavour! Rice water, the ancient Asian beauty elixir, is no longer just used to nourish grains.

It's about to become the secret ingredient in your skincare routine, offering a gentle yet effective way to transform your skin. But how can you seamlessly incorporate this ancient wisdom into your modern routine? Let's embark on the journey of rice water metallurgy!

The Cleaning Caper: Double Duty Delight: Instead of a regular cleanser, choose a gentle, natural cleanser and mix it with cold rice water. Imagine rice water acting like a soothing mist, soothing your skin while the cleanser draws out impurities.
Rinse off and enjoy a refreshing, balanced feeling. Micellar Magic: Micellar water fan? Upgrade it with rice water! Mix equal parts Micellar water and rice water and soak a cotton pad.
Apply evenly on the face and discover the dual cleansing power of micelles and the brightening properties of rice water. Invigorating Symphony: Unexpected Spritz: Ditch the harsh tonics and embrace the refreshing feeling of rice water mist.

Fill a spray bottle with cold rice water and lightly spray it on your face after washing your face. This energises the skin, balances pH levels and prepares the skin for serum or moisturiser. Imagine the drops of rice water settling like tiny pearls, nourishing your skin.

Mask Mania: Turn your favourite mask into mixed rice! Instead of water, use rice water to activate your clay or sheet mask. Imagine the nutrients from the rice water seeping into the mask, amplifying its benefits and leaving your skin pampered and nourished.

Beyond the basics: DIY fun: Don't just use rice water, get creative with it! Mix it with honey for a hydrating face mask, aloe vera for soothing properties, or turmeric for a glow boost. Think of your kitchen as a beauty laboratory, experimenting with different combinations to personalise your routine.

Happy Bath Bonus: Add leftover rice water to your bath for a luxurious bath. Imagine the soothing properties of rice water enveloping your body, leaving your skin soft and glowing.

Remember: Consistency is key! Incorporating rice water into your routine regularly will unleash its full potential. However, listen to your skin and adjust frequency or method as needed.

Embrace the journey: Think of rice water not as a trend but as a reconnection with ancient wisdom. With a little creativity and a little rice water, you can turn your current routine into a nourishing ritual that celebrates your unique beauty. So get out, explore and witness the rice water revolution! As transformation begins at your fingertips, embrace the ancient magic and let your skin shine!

Chapter 10

Beyond the blush: Rice water's journey from face to body bloom Rice water, the humble kitchen staple, steps out of the guard - eats and finds himself in the spotlight - but not just for your face!
This ancient elixir spreads its wings, delivering a host of benefits to your hair and body, promising a transformation from head to toe. So, ditch the chemical cocktails and enjoy the natural magic of rice water!

Harmonious hair: Say goodbye to split ends: Imagine your hair is like a strand of silk, easily broken. Rice water, with its amino acids and proteins, acts as a gentle conditioner, strengthening hair strands and saying goodbye to split ends.

Rinse your hair with rice water after shampooing and imagine it absorbing good nutrients for your hair, making it soft and easy to manage.

Embrace the bounce: Is your hair limp and lifeless? The inositol content in rice water acts like a little magician, plumping up hair strands and increasing volume.

After shampooing, massage rice water into your scalp and hair, imagining it is infusing life into each strand. Wash it off and witness the voluptuous transformation!

Natural Shine Enhancer: Forget about oily products! The natural sugars in rice water coat your hair, reflecting light and adding healthy shine without weighing it down. After the final rinse, use rice water as a leave-in treatment, imagining it polishing your hair to a silky shine.

Bodily Happiness: Soothing Soak: Imagine a bath of warm water mixed with rice water, its soothing properties enveloping your body.

The starch content acts as a gentle emollient, soothing irritated skin and leaving it soft and supple. Add rice water to the bath and imagine your worries melting away like grains of rice, leaving you relaxed and rejuvenated.

Fun exfoliator: Mix rice water with oatmeal or coffee grounds to create a natural body scrub. Massage gently into skin, imagining softening and exfoliating rice water that will remove dullness, leaving skin smooth, radiant. Rinse off and enjoy your revitalised skin.

After-sun lollipop: Are sunburns bringing you down? The refreshing properties of rice water will come to your rescue! Dip a towel in cold rice water and apply it to the sunburned area, imagining that the cool compress will soothe the irritation and promote healing.

Consistency is key! Using rice water regularly for hair and body will maximise its potential. However, listen to your skin and hair's needs and adjust frequency or method as needed.

Bonus tip : Don't throw away leftover rice! Use it as a body scrub or mix it into your compost bin for lasting effects. So, open your pantry and unleash the transformative power of rice water!

With a little creativity and a dash of ancient wisdom, you can nourish your hair and body from head to toe, achieving radiant, all-around skin. Remember, beauty begins with your fingertips, so embrace the rice revolution and let your inner and outer beauty flourish!

1.From grain to glory: Unleash the revitalization of rice water for hair and scalp Moves, chemical cocktails and harsh treatments! The secret to silky hair and a healthy scalp lies in a pantry staple: rice water . This ancient elixir, used by Asian cultures for centuries, is ready to be your new hair hero, delivering a natural, gentle and effective approach to achieving hair nirvana.

Embrace the hairstyle: Samurai assassin with split ends: Imagine your hair strands like those of warriors, prone to breakage. Rice water, rich in amino acids and proteins, acts as a gentle conditioner, strengthening each strand of hair from root to tip.

Rinse your hair with rice water after shampooing, imagining that your hair will absorb nutrients and become stronger with each wash. Say goodbye to split ends and hello to soft, smooth, manageable hair!

Goddess Ritual Episode: Does your hair lack the bounce of a lively clown? The inositol content in rice water acts like a small miracle worker, volumizing hair strands and increasing volume like a magic potion. After shampooing, massage rice water into your scalp and hair, imagining it is infusing life into each strand. Rinse and witness the transformation: soft strands become bouncy and full of life!

Shine like a star: Forget fatty products! The natural sugars in rice water coat your hair, reflecting light and adding healthy shine without weighing it down. After the final rinse, use rice water as a leave-in treatment, imagining it polishing your hair to a silky shine. Imagine your hair shining like a star under the spotlight without harsh chemicals.

Symphony of scalp serenity: Soothes itchy skin: Does a dry, itchy scalp make you feel like a grumpy troll? The gentle properties of rice water will come to your rescue! Its mild astringent properties help balance the pH of the scalp, while its anti-inflammatory properties help soothe irritation.

After shampooing, massage cold rice water into your scalp, imagining it will soothe discomfort and restore peace to your scalp.

Dandruff treatment:

Is dandruff bothering your journey? Don't worry, rice water can be your knight in shining armor! Its antifungal properties help fight the dandruff-causing Malassezia fungus, keeping your scalp healthy and dandruff-free.

Wash your hair regularly with rice water, imagining that it helps eliminate dandruff and restores the natural balance to your scalp.

Stimulates a Garden of Growth: Imagine your scalp as a fertile garden where hair follicles grow like tiny seedlings.

Rice water is rich in B vitamins and minerals that can act as a natural fertiliser, stimulating hair growth and promoting a healthy environment for the scalp. Incorporate washing your hair with rice water regularly into your routine, imagining that it nourishes your hair follicles and encourages them to grow.

Remember: Consistency is key! Using rice water regularly for your hair and scalp will maximize its potential. However, listen to your hair's needs and adjust the frequency or method as needed.

Bonus tip : Don't throw away leftover rice! Use it as a body scrub or compost it for a sustainable feel. So, open your pantry and unleash the transformative power of rice water!

With a little creativity and a little ancient wisdom, you can naturally achieve silky smooth hair and a healthy scalp. Remember, the journey to hair nirvana starts with simple ingredients and a commitment to nourishing hair from the roots. Enjoy the renaissance of rice water and let your hair shine like a real star!

2.From rice fields to relaxation rituals: Immerse yourself in the calm waters of a rice water bath. Throw away salt baths and bubble baths! Today we begin our peaceful journey, guided by the humble yet powerful magic of rice water. Imagine your bathtub transformed into a haven of relaxation, where the gentle caress of rice water soothes your body and mind.

As you gather your ingredients and get ready to experience the ultimate self-care ritual. The Soothing Symphony: The Milky Serenity: Prepare a pot of rice water, imagine it is absorbing the essence of the rice grain as it boils. Imagine its milky white colour turning your bath water into a tranquil nutrient pool. Pour it in, letting the steam carry the soothing aroma.

Blooming flowers: Enhance the experience with the feeling of nature. Scattering rose petals, lavender buds or chamomile in water, visualising their colors and scents will add to the sensory journey. Imagine them infusing water with their healing properties. A soothing companion: Don't forget the essentials!

Light soothing scented candles, dim the lights, and turn on soothing music. Create an atmosphere that invites deep relaxation, letting your worries melt away like grains of rice dissolving in water. Outside the bath:

Foot sanctuary: Treat your hard-working feet to an exclusive ritual. Fill a basin with warm rice water and add a few drops of essential oils such as peppermint or eucalyptus. Imagine water enveloping your feet, soothing pain and leaving them feeling refreshed and revitalised.

Delight Exfoliator: Mix rice water with ground oatmeal or coffee grounds to gently exfoliate. Massage it onto your feet, imagining soft rice water and the scrub will remove dead skin cells, revealing smooth, radiant skin. Rinse off and reward yourself with a new feeling as consistency is key!

Regularly incorporating rice water into your bathing routine will reap its benefits. However, listen to your skin and adjust frequency or method as needed.

Bonus tip : Don't throw away leftover rice! Use it to make a delicious meal or compost it to create a sense of sustainability. So, open your pantry and unlock the transformative power of rice water. With a little creativity and a little self-care, you can transform your bathtub or foot bath into a peaceful haven.

Remember, relaxation is a journey, not a destination. Immerse yourself in the soothing waters of rice water and let its gentle magic wash away stress, leaving you feeling refreshed and invigorated.

Part 4

Beyond beauty: Integrate sustainability and ethics into your rice water ritual As we explore the magic of rice water for skin, hair and body, we don't forget the bigger picture. Sustainability and ethical considerations should be woven into our beauty routines, like the threads of a vibrant tapestry. So, before you begin your rice water sourcing journey, take a moment to reflect:

Symphony of Sustainability: Conscious Sourcing: Choose rice grown with sustainable measures, such as using water in an organic or environmentally friendly way. Imagine rice fields full of life, cultivated with respect for the environment. Remember, healthy ecosystems create healthy ingredients.

Recycle and reuse: Don't throw away leftover rice! Cook it as usual, knowing that its nutrients have been partially extracted from your beauty potion. Or compost to feed your garden, creating a beautiful closed loop.

Less is more: Avoid using too much rice water, especially if you live in places where water is scarce. Choose concentrated infusions or use them strategically in your routine. Remember, conscious consumption is the key to a sustainable future.

Ethical Equation: Focus on Fair Trade: Find rice water products from brands that support fair trade practices, ensuring fair wages and working conditions for farmers . Imagine the smiles on their faces knowing that their hard work contributes to a more equitable world.

Local Love: If possible, buy rice locally to reduce transportation emissions and support your community. Think of it as voting for your local farmer and reducing your carbon footprint.

Cruelty-Free Pledge: Choose brands that are cruelty-free and do not test their products on animals. Imagine playful animals frolicking freely, knowing that your beauty choices align with your compassion.

Remember: Sustainability and ethical considerations are not just trends but essential elements of a responsible beauty routine. By making conscious choices, you can contribute to a healthier planet and a more equitable world, while enjoying the benefits of rice water.

Embrace the journey: Think of your rice water ritual as an opportunity to connect with nature, support ethical practices, and minimise your impact on the environment.

With each conscious choice, you will create a ripple effect of positive change, both internally and externally. As you go ahead to explore, remember: beauty and sustainability go hand in hand in the rice water revolution! Let your inner and outer light shine through the power of conscious care.

Chapter 11

From Grain to Wonderfulness: Choosing Rice with Awareness in Your Rice Water Custom Rice water, the humble solution of magnificence, holds covered up profundities past its skin-soothing enchantment.
As we set out on this journey of change, let's dive more profound and guarantee our rice water custom reverberates with obligation, both for ourselves and the planet. Choosing rice shrewdly isn't almost aesthetics; it's almost grasping a all encompassing approach to excellence.

The Sourcing Orchestra: Organic Concordance: Envision your skin lolling within the delicate touch of rice developed without hurtful chemicals. Choose natural rice, free from pesticides and fertilisers, imagining dynamic areas abounding with life, not hurtful buildups.

Keep in mind, sound soil nurtures healthy rice, which in turn feeds your skin. Water-Wise Waltz: Water shortage may be a squeezing concern. Select rice developed with maintainable water administration hones, like rain-fed farming or productive water system frameworks.

Envision the rice areas flourishing without draining valuable assets, guaranteeing a future where magnificence customs do not come at the taking a toll of natural strain. Nearby Adore Number:
Back your community and minimise your carbon impression by choosing locally sourced rice. Picture the rice travelling a shorter distance, diminishing transportation emanations and supporting nearby ranchers. Keep in mind, each cognizant choice swells outwards, making a more economical excellence community.

The Natural Condition: Differences Move: Biodiversity is key to a solid planet. Pick rice assortments developed in different environments, supporting local plants and creatures that contribute to a balanced environment.

Envision the rice areas buzzing with life, a sanctuary for pollinators and animals alike, guaranteeing the sensitive web of nature remains vibrant. Reasonable Exchange Celebration: Celebrate moral hones by choosing rice sourced through reasonable exchange activities.

Envision the grins on farmers' faces, knowing their difficult work is remunerated with reasonable compensation and working conditions. Keep in mind, magnificence ceremonies ought to engage, not misuse, the communities that maintain them. Waste Not,

Need Not: Minimise your affect by maintaining a strategic distance from intemperate rice utilisation and composting extra rice. Picture the grains being renewed as nutrient-rich soil, feeding your plant and completing a lovely circle of life. Keep in mind, cognizant utilisation is key to a maintainable future.

Grasp the Travel: Each cognizant choice you make in sourcing your rice water is a step towards a more excellent world, both interior and out. Let your rice water custom be a celebration of duty, a confirmation to your commitment to an economical future.

With each careful scoop, you make a swell impact of positive change, guaranteeing that your excellence journey aligns with the well-being of our planet and its individuals.
So, go forward, investigate, and keep in mind – choosing rice responsibly is the primary step in your rice water transformation! Let your inward and external shine transmit with the control of conscious care.

From grain to glory: Turning rice water into a zero-waste ritual Rice water, an essential ingredient in the humble kitchen, enters the landscape, offering softness yet strength.

But don't forget that beauty shouldn't come at the expense of our planet! So turn your rice water drinking ritual into a zero-waste celebration, where every grain counts and sustainability is the focus. Wasteful waltz: Measure twice, brew once:

Take the guesswork out of it, use a measuring cup to avoid over-stirring the rice, ensuring every grain gets the job done. Imagine the leftover rice laughing its way out of the pot, ready for its next adventure.

Upcycle: Don't throw away cooked rice! Use it in stir-fries, soups or even to make crispy rice cakes. Think of it as a culinary makeover, giving rice a second life to nourish your body and wallet.

Final compost: Leftover rice water is not worth draining! Give it a major role in your compost bin. Imagine it nourishing your garden, returning essential nutrients to the earth, and completing a beautiful cycle of life.

Supporting sustainable symphonies: Organic harmony: Choose organic rice, free of harmful chemicals and pesticides. Imagine vibrant fields full of life, where rice grows in harmony with nature and its purity is expressed through your beauty ritual.

Water-Wise Waltz: Choose rice grown using sustainable water management practices. Imagine fields that thrive without depleting precious resources, ensuring a future where beauty rituals do not cause water scarcity.

Fair Trade Festival: Celebrate ethical practices by choosing rice from fair trade initiatives. Imagine the smiles on the faces of farmers knowing that their hard work contributes to a more equitable and sustainable world.

Remember, your beauty choices can empower your community and protect the environment. Beyond Ritual: Consider reducing waste and supporting sustainable practices as the foundation of your rice water journey. Let each conscious choice radiate outward, creating a wave of positive chang

DIY Delight: Harness the power of DIY! Instead of buying pre-made rice water, make your own from leftover rice. Imagine the satisfaction of creating your beauty elixir from scratch and knowing exactly what's in it.

Spread the word: Share your zero-waste rice water ritual with friends and family. Inspire them to join the eco-friendly beauty movement, creating a collective impact that goes beyond your own halo. Shop with a purpose: Support brands that prioritize sustainability and ethical practices.

Let your spending power speak volumes about your worth, encouraging positive change in the beauty industry by Embracing sustainability does not mean sacrificing results.

It's about making conscious choices that benefit your skin, the planet, and the people who bring this ancient elixir to your doorstep. So go ahead, explore, and remember: the zero-waste ritual of drinking rice water is a beautiful act of self-love and care for the planet. Let your inner and outer radiance shine with the power of conscious beauty.

1.Beyond Broth: Decoding the magic of recycling leftover rice Leftover rice: the silent protagonist of countless meals, often placed in the back of the refrigerator, destined to die alone. But what if I told you that this humble grain holds the key to culinary creativity and sustainable living? Imagine turning your leftover rice into a symphony of delicious flavors, minimising waste and igniting your kitchen's inner alchemist!

The Upcycling Odyssey: Crispy Bread Festival: Don't let the mushy rice get you down! Mash it with herbs, spices and cheese, form bite-sized balls and cover with a crispy panko crust. Imagine them sizzling in the pan, transformed into golden nuggets of joy, ready to be dipped in your favourite sauce.

Overlooked Symphony: Let your imagination run wild! Mix leftover rice with colourful vegetables, leftover proteins, and flavorful sauces. Imagine the wok dancing with vibrant colours, creating a stir-fry masterpiece that is both delicious and environmentally friendly.

Rice Cake Caper: Think beyond the store-bought version! Spread leftover rice thinly on a baking sheet, bake until crispy, and sprinkle with your favourite toppings.

Imagine creating delicious rice cakes for dipping, sweet rice cakes drizzled with honey, or even delicious pizza-style rice cakes filled with cheese and vegetables.

Stuffed Fiesta peppers: Core peppers, stuff with mixed rice and bake until tender. Imagine peppers transformed into colorful treasure chests, bursting with flavour and showing off your recycling prowess.

Soup Surprise: Don't let leftover rice become a one-note affair! Add a little coconut milk, a squeeze of lime and fresh herbs for a Thai-inspired dish. Or turn it into a creamy tomato soup with a little pesto. Remember that imagination is the only limit!

Beyond the Plate: Beauty Potion: Did you know that leftover rice water is a secret weapon for your skin and hair? Mix it, filter it and use it as a toner, hair conditioner or even a mask! Imagine your leftover rice doing double duty, nourishing both your body and your beauty routine.

Compost Crusader: Don't throw away that leftover rice! Add them to your compost bin, where they will decompose into nutrient-rich soil, ready to nourish your garden and complete the cycle of life. Remember: Upcycling is more than just a trend; it is a celebration of ingenuity and creativity.

With every grain processed, you reduce waste, inspire culinary joy, and contribute to a more sustainable future. So embrace the spirit of recycling, unleash your inner kitchen alchemist, and discover the hidden magic of leftover rice!

Chapter 12

Beyond Rice Water: Cultivate an Ethical Beauty Garden Your journey to glowing skin and a healthy planet goes beyond what's in your pantry. While rice water is a wonderful tool for personal transformation, true beauty flourishes when we cultivate an ecosystem of ethical practices that extend beyond individual actions. Let's get out of the toilet and into the wider world, where our voices can become collective whispers, weaving a tapestry of change.

From Seed to Unity: Amplify the Whispers: Share your love of ethical beauty with friends and family. Educate them about the impact of their choices, encourage them to join the movement.
Imagine your knowledge flourishing in a collective conversation, empowering others to make informed decisions. Seedling Support: Find brands that prioritise ethical sourcing, fair business practices and sustainable production.

Look for certifications and do your research, be a savvy consumer who votes with your wallet. Imagine these brands thriving like healthy seedlings, nurtured by your support.
Speak up: Don't hesitate to speak up tha will Reach out to your favourite brands, expressing your desire for transparency and ethical practices.

Join online communities and advocacy groups, amplifying the collective voice of conscious consumers and your voice joining a chorus, demanding change and pushing the industry towards a more responsible future.

Sow the seeds of change: Volunteer your time or skills with organisations that work to promote ethical beauty practices. Help them develop educational initiatives, raise awareness, or even advocate for policy changes.

Imagine your efforts towards a better future where ethical beauty is not just a trend but also the norm that We are not individual islands but interconnected parts of a larger ecosystem. Our actions, no matter how small, can spread outward and create positive change.

Let your commitment to ethical beauty be more than a personal mission; whether it is a call to action, an invitation to cultivate a garden of ethical practices that nourish both ourselves and the planet. Join the movement:

Share your story: Inspire others by sharing your ethical beauty journey on social media or on your blog. Start the conversation: Host a meetup or focus group in your community to raise awareness about ethical beauty practices.

Support ethical brands: Make a conscious effort to buy from brands that align with your values. Advocates for Change: Contact your representatives and urge them to support policies that promote sustainable and ethical beauty practices.

Together, we can create a world where beauty shines not just on our faces but at the heart of our industries and the prosperity of our planet. Join the chorus and watch the beautiful virtuous garden bloom!

1.Beyond the label: Discover the hidden gems of ethical beauty In the dazzling world of beauty products, the allure of quirky packaging and trendy ingredients can dazzle. But what if we told you that the real magic lies beneath the surface, in the hidden stories of responsible sourcing?

Join us on our journey to discover brands that go beyond glitz and glamour, integrating sustainability and ethics into the very fabric of their products. Imagine a world where: Sparkling mica does not sparkle with the tears of child labour.

Instead, it comes from ethical mines that prioritise worker safety and fair wages. Luxury oil leaves no trace of deforestation. They come from farms that nurture biodiversity and support local communities.

Exotic ingredients not extracted from their natural habitat. They are grown sustainably while respecting the delicate balance of our planet. Become an ethical beauty alchemist:

Unmask hidden heroes: Don't just rely on flashy brands. Look for brands that prioritise ethical sourcing, fair trade, and sustainable practices. Look for certifications like Fairtrade, B Corp and FSC.

Become a label detective: Check the ingredient list. Avoid brands that use ingredients that are unethically sourced or cause damage to the environment.

Look for brands that disclose their sourcing practices transparently. Join the Ethical Beauty Tribe: Connect with online communities and advocacy groups that promote ethical beauty. Share your knowledge and inspire others to make conscious choices.

Supporting Changemakers: Choose brands that lead by example. Invest in products that align with your values, even if it means spending a little more. Remember, your purchasing power is a powerful vote for change. Beyond personal action:

Amplifying whispers: Share your love for ethical beauty with friends and family. Educate them about the impact of their choices and encourage them to join the movement.

Speak up: Don't be afraid to speak up! Contact brands and express your desire for transparency and ethical practices. Participate in online campaigns and advocacy efforts.

Sow the seeds of change: Volunteer your time or skills with organisations that work to promote ethical beauty practices. Help them develop educational initiatives, raise awareness, or even advocate for policy changes.

Remember: True beauty flourishes not just on our skin but at the heart of our industries and the prosperity of our planet. By supporting brands with responsible sourcing practices, you become a co-creator of a more sustainable and ethical future.

Let your conscious choices radiate outward, transforming your beautiful landscape into a responsible garden. Join the movement: Share your ethical beauty discoveries online.

Organise an evening to socialise with friends and support sustainable brands. Start a petition or write to your favourite brand demanding transparency and ethical sourcing.

Supports organisations working to promote ethical beauty practices. Together, we can rewrite the history of beauty, one responsible choice at a time. Let's discover the real gems, not only on our faces but also in the world around us!

Conclusion

1.Rice water renaissance: A roundup of glowing skin and sustainable options Ah, rice water! This humble staple reveals its hidden depths, offering a natural, gentle and effective approach to achieving skin nirvana. As we close this chapter on the ritual of drinking rice water, let's collect the pearls of wisdom and imagine the hidden benefits that await you:

Because your skin will be refreshed: Hydration Hero: Rice water, rich in starch and amino acids, acts as a moisture magnet, leaving your skin plump and dewy. Imagine it quenching your skin's thirst, leaving it soft and supple.

Soothing Saviour: Say goodbye to discomfort! The anti-inflammatory properties of rice water can soothe eczema, rashes and even sunburn, helping to soothe and restore comfort to your skin.

Brightening Bard: Do you want radiant skin? The inositol content in rice water can help reduce hyperpigmentation and skin darkening, resulting in brighter, more even skin tone. Imagine it eliminating dullness and revealing your inner light.

Scalp Serenity: Don't forget your scalp!

The antifungal properties of rice water can fight the dandruff-causing Malassezia fungus, while its gentle astringent properties help balance the pH of the scalp, creating a healthy environment for hair to grow. Imagine it nourishing your scalp and creating a haven for strong, healthy hair.

Beyond Benefits: Sustainability Symphony: Choose locally sourced organic rice and reduce waste by recycling leftover rice or composting it. Imagine being part of a harmonious cycle that nourishes your skin and respects the planet.

Ethical Equation: Supports brands that prioritize fair trade practices and ethical sourcing, ensuring beauty choices align with your values. Imagine your rice water drinking ritual contributing to a more just and equitable world.

Conscious Consumption: Take a "less is more" approach, using rice water strategically and choosing reusable containers. Imagine your bathroom becoming a haven of sustainability, where beauty rituals are intertwined with environmental responsibility.

Consistency is key! Incorporating rice water into your routine regularly will unleash its full potential. Listen to your skin's needs and adjust frequency or method as needed. So are you ready to embark on the rice water revival?

Let this ancient elixir be your guide, leading you to radiant skin, a sustainable future, and a more conscious approach to beauty. Remember, you have the power to cultivate both external and internal radiance, one conscious choice at a time!

2.Beauty beyond the bottle: Building a sustainable skin care mecca Forget crowded shelves and endless aisles! Sustainable skin care is not about sacrifice, but about weaving self-care with intention and responsibility. Imagine you are a skilled artisan, creating a beauty routine that nourishes both your skin and the planet.

Embrace the alchemy of less: Declare with compassion: Befriend your hairdresser's "KonMari Method." Thank each product for its service, then release these unused wonders with a trade, donation or responsible recycling. Remember, less can be more, especially when it comes to impact.

Multitasking Wonders: One-use Wonders in the Ditch! Look for products that can be used for multiple purposes, such as a cream blush that doubles as a lip tint or a conditioner that works for both face and hair. Imagine your makeup bag transformed into a multi-purpose treasure chest.

Refills and Reuse Revolution: Choose refillable options or invest in reusable utensils and containers. Imagine your bathroom becoming a haven of sustainability, where waste takes a back seat to conscious choices.

DIY Delight: Harness the power of DIY! Discover natural ingredients and simple recipes to create your own beauty blends. Imagine yourself in the position of an alchemist in the kitchen, mixing personalised potions with minimal impact on the environment.

Outside the bathroom: Water warrior: Minimise water consumption in your routine. Choose shorter showers, use water-efficient showerheads, and collect rainwater for washing. Imagine that each drop saved becomes a ripple of change.

Packaging pioneers: Find brands that prioritise sustainable packaging and reduce plastic waste. Look for certifications like FSC and recycled materials. Remember, your purchasing power is a vote for change.

Ingredient Integrity: Choose natural and organic ingredients whenever possible. Avoid products with harsh chemicals or microplastics. Imagine your skin thanking you for nourishing it with nature's goodness.

Ethical Advocates: Supports brands that prioritise fair trade practices and responsible sourcing which show that beauty should not come at the expense of exploitation. Remember: True beauty flourishes not just on your skin but at the heart of our industries and the prosperity of our planet.

By adopting responsible and sustainable practices, you become a co-creator of a better future. Let your conscious choices radiate outward, transforming the skin care landscape into a tapestry woven with respect for the environment and ourselves.

Join the movement: Share your sustainable skin care tips online. Host a "less is more" exchange party with friends. Start a petition or write to your favourite brand to demand sustainable practices. Support organisations working for ethical and sustainable beauty.

Together, we can rewrite the history of beauty, one conscious choice at a time. Let's paint a picture of a more sustainable future, where beauty not only shines on our faces but also shines in the world around us.

3.Beyond Grains and Splinters: The unique skin journey you've been waiting for As we say goodbye to the world of rice water and sustainable skin care, remember that it's not the end but a beautiful start.

Your journey to healthy, radiant skin is unique, and while rice water offers an appealing path, it's just one step in your personal adventure. Remember: Customization is key: What works for one person may not work for another.

Listen to your skin, test different methods, and consult with a trusted dermatologist to create a personalised plan that addresses your needs and concerns. your particular mind. Dermatologists: Wise guides for your skin: Think of dermatologists as skin health alchemists.

They have the knowledge and expertise to decode your skin's language, diagnose potential problems, and recommend treatments tailored to your needs. Don't hesitate to ask for their advice, especially if you have concerns or need professional advice.

Total harmony: True beauty goes beyond the surface. Remember, healthy skin often reflects a healthy lifestyle. Nourish your body with balanced meals, prioritise good sleep, and effectively manage stress. These holistic practices will complement your skin care routine and contribute to your overall health. So as you begin the next chapter in your skin's journey: Experiment: Explore different ingredients, techniques and philosophies. Remember that discovery is an essential part of the journey.

Get expert advice: Don't be afraid to consult a dermatologist. They can be your trusted allies in navigating the vast world of skin care.

Celebrate your individuality: Your skin is a unique canvas and your personalised approach to skin care is a celebration of that uniqueness. May your skin journey be filled with self-discovery, radiant results, and the profound realisation that true beauty lies in following your unique path.

Appendix

Glossary of terms related to rice water and skin care. Additional sources and research references. Decoding the language of rice water and skin care: A cool glossary Welcome intrepid beauty explorer! As you venture into the exciting realm of rice water and skin care, fear not! This quirky glossary will be your trusted guide, translating terms and revealing the secrets hidden in each term.

Rice water: Infusion: The elixir you create by soaking rice in water, releasing nutrients that benefit the skin. Imagine little fairies dancing inside, unleashing their beauty magic.

Starch: The main ingredient found in rice water, acts as a moisture magnet, helping your skin become plump and moisturised. Think of it as a smooth cloud, gently hydrating your parched skin.

Amino acids: Building blocks of protein, found in abundance in rice water. Think of them as tiny construction workers rebuilding and strengthening the skin barrier.

Fermented rice water: Rice water contains good bacteria, known to soothe irritation and improve skin texture. Think of it as a bubbly champagne toast for your skin, sparkling with beneficial probiotics.

Skin care: Hydration: The key to healthy, happy skin. Think of it as a way to quench your skin's thirst, leaving it soft and bright like a well-watered garden. Anti-inflammatory: Properties soothe irritated skin, like a gentle breeze after a sunburn. Think of it as a soothing melody, soothing redness and discomfort.

Brightener: Ingredients help reduce hyperpigmentation and even skin tone, bringing bright skin from within. Think of it as a gentle brushstroke, removing dullness and revealing your natural glow.

Scalp: The ecosystem that nourishes your hair is often forgotten. Rice water can help fight dandruff and balance the pH of the scalp, creating a healthy environment for strong locks. Think of it as fertile soil, nurturing your glorious roots.

Sustainability: Choose practices that minimise environmental impact, such as using locally sourced rice and composting excess water. Think of it as dancing with Mother Nature, honouring her generosity and leaving a gentle mark.

Ethical Sourcing: Ensures fair wages and working conditions for those involved in the production of beauty products. Think of it as a respectful handshake, connecting you to the people who bring these ingredients to life.

Remember: This glossary is just a starting point! Explore, experiment and discover what works best for your unique skin. And most of all, have fun on your journey to radiant, lasting beauty! Additional resources and research references.

Beyond the glossary: Revealing the treasures of the Beauty Library Your quest for knowledge doesn't end here, intrepid explorer! Consider this your map to a deeper understanding of rice water, sustainable skin care, and the fascinating world of beauty.

For the Rice Whisperer: Delve into the archives: Explore ancient texts and historical documents to understand the origins and traditional uses of rice water in different cultures . Imagine yourself as the Indiana Jones of skin care, uncovering the secrets of our ancestors.

Science Detective: Dive into research articles and clinical studies to better understand the scientific evidence behind the benefits of rice water. Imagine you're a scientist in a lab coat, unravelling the mysteries of its composition.

DIY Delights: Explore blogs, online communities, and recipe books dedicated to creating your own rice water recipes. Imagine you're an alchemist in the kitchen, concocting personalised elixirs using natural ingredients.

Sustainable Skin Care Mecca: Eco-Warriors Unite: Join online forums and organisations dedicated to sustainable beauty practices. Imagine connecting with a global community of like-minded people, sharing advice and advocating for change. Certification Compass: Decipher the maze of sustainability certifications like Fair Trade, B Corp and FSC. Think of these seals as guiding stars, leading you to brands that align with your values.

Documentaries & Films: Immerse yourself in documentaries and films that explore the environmental impact of the beauty industry and inspire sustainable solutions.being transported to different parts of the world and witnessing the challenges and innovations shaping the future of beauty.

Beyond Skin Deep: Total Harmony: Explore the connection between skin health and overall wellness. Discover the impact diet, sleep and stress have on your skin. Imagine you're a total detective, piecing together the puzzle of radiant health.

Dialogue with a dermatologist: Don't hesitate to seek expert advice! Consult a dermatologist for personalised advice on incorporating rice water or other remedies into your skin care routine. Think of them as your skin's wise advisors, offering expert advice and personalised recommendations.

Show off your personality: Remember that your skin journey is unique! What works for one person may not work for another. Embrace your personality and experiment with different methods to discover what makes your skin tick and This is just a glimpse of the vast world of resources available. Be curious, explore with an open mind and above all, enjoy the journey towards a radiant being, both inside and out!